THE ULTIMATE
DIABETIC
AIR FRYER
COOKBOOK
for BEGINNERS

*Elevate Your Health with a Cookbook Filled with Nutrient-Rich
Recipes and Expert Guidance for Balanced Living*

Isabella Abrams

Contents

CHAPTER 5.
PORK RECIPES 67

CHAPTER 6.
BEEF RECIPES 74

LAMB RECIPES 79

CHAPTER 7.
FISH RECIPES 84

SEAFOOD RECIPES 91

INTRODUCTION

Welcome to the Diabetic Air Fryer Cookbook for Beginners, a comprehensive guide to cooking delicious and healthy meals that cater to individuals with diabetes. If you're reading this, chances are you're someone who has struggled to find the right balance between managing diabetes and maintaining a healthy diet. You're not alone – many people with diabetes struggle to find tasty meal options that won't spike their blood sugar levels.

But don't worry – you've come to the right place. This cookbook is designed to provide you with easy-to-follow recipes that are both nutritious and flavorful, all while keeping your blood sugar levels in check. By the end of this book, you'll have the tools you need to make delicious meals that will make your taste buds sing and your body feel great.

As a chef and nutritionist with years of experience, I understand the challenges that come with managing diabetes. That's why I've put together this cookbook, drawing from my extensive knowledge of nutrition and my passion for creating wholesome, tasty dishes. I'm excited to share my expertise with you and help you make positive changes to your diet and lifestyle.

In the following chapters, you'll find a wide range of recipes that will cater to your dietary needs, including breakfast dishes, snacks, main courses, and desserts. With each recipe, I'll provide you with detailed nutritional information, so you can make informed choices about what you eat. You'll also find helpful tips on how to use your air fryer effectively, so you can get the most out of this versatile kitchen appliance.

By following the recipes and tips in this book, you'll not only be able to manage your diabetes effectively but also enjoy a wider range of flavorful and healthy meals. So let's get started! In the first chapter, we'll go over some basics of cooking with an air fryer, and then we'll jump right into some mouth-watering recipes that you won't be able to resist.

What is an Air Fryer?

An air fryer is a kitchen appliance that cooks food by circulating hot air around it, similar to a convection oven. It uses little to no oil to cook the food, making it a healthier alternative to traditional frying methods. The hot air circulates around the food, creating a crispy outer layer while keeping the inside moist and tender. Air fryers can be used to cook a variety of foods, including meats, vegetables, and even desserts. They are often compact and easy to use, making them a popular appliance in many households.

Why Should the Diabetic Use an Air Fryer?

Diabetic individuals can benefit from using an air fryer for several reasons:

Healthier Cooking Method: An air fryer uses little to no oil, making it a healthier alternative to traditional frying methods. This means that the food cooked in an air fryer is lower in fat and calories, which is important for individuals with diabetes who need to watch their weight.

Lower Glycemic Index: Foods that are cooked in an air fryer tend to have a lower glycemic index compared to those that are deep-fried. This means that they are less likely to cause a spike in blood sugar levels, which is important for individuals with diabetes who need to control their blood sugar.

Versatility: An air fryer can be used to cook a variety of foods, including meats, vegetables, and even desserts. This versatility allows individuals with diabetes to enjoy a wide range of healthy and flavorful meals.

Convenience: An air fryer is often compact and easy to use, making it a convenient appliance for individuals with diabetes who may have limited time or mobility. The quick cooking time also means that meals can be prepared quickly and easily, which is important for individuals with busy lifestyles.

An air fryer is a great cooking appliance for individuals with diabetes as it offers a healthier and convenient way to prepare a variety of foods while keeping blood sugar levels in check.

Tips for why you should use an Air Fryer

- Preheating is optional, but some people find it helpful to ensure even cooking.
- To keep your meals healthier, use a minimal amount of oil or use a spray-on oil from a reusable bottle.
- Shake the basket halfway through cooking to ensure even cooking.
- Cooking times may vary depending on the food, so it's best to keep an eye on it and adjust accordingly.
- Avoid overcrowding the basket to allow hot air to circulate around the food and ensure even cooking.
- To prevent sticking, you can use parchment paper or tin foil.

Tips on how to take care of it

1. **Clean it regularly:** After each use, allow the air fryer to cool down, then clean it thoroughly. You can do this by removing the basket and pan and washing them with soap and water. The exterior of the air fryer can be wiped down with a damp cloth.

2. **Do not use abrasive cleaners:** Avoid using abrasive cleaners or scrubbers on the air fryer as they can damage the non-stick coating.

3. **Do not submerge the air fryer in water:** The electrical components of the air fryer should not be exposed to water, so do not submerge it in water or place it in a dishwasher.

4. **Use the correct accessories:** Only use accessories that are specifically designed for your air fryer. Using incompatible accessories can cause damage to the air fryer or affect its performance.

5. **Store it properly:** When not in use, store the air fryer in a cool and dry place, away from moisture and heat sources.

6. **Check for signs of wear and tear:** Regularly inspect your air fryer for signs of wear and tear, such as cracks or scratches. If you notice any damage, stop using the air fryer and contact the manufacturer for repair or replacement.

By following these tips, you can ensure that your air fryer lasts for a long time and continues to work effectively.

What is Diabetes?

Diabetes is a chronic medical condition that affects how your body processes blood sugar (glucose). Glucose is an essential source of energy for your body, but when you have diabetes, your body either can't produce enough insulin (a hormone that regulates blood sugar levels) or can't effectively use the insulin it produces. As a result, your blood sugar levels can become too high, which can cause a variety of health problems.

There are two main types of diabetes:

Type 1 diabetes: This is an autoimmune disease in which the body's immune system attacks and destroys the cells in the pancreas that produce insulin. Type 1 diabetes is usually diagnosed in children and young adults, and it requires lifelong insulin therapy.

Type 2 diabetes: This is the most common form of diabetes, and it usually develops in adults. In type 2 diabetes, the body becomes resistant to insulin or doesn't produce enough insulin to regulate blood sugar levels. Type 2 diabetes can often be managed through diet, exercise, and medication.

Diabetes can cause a range of complications if left untreated, including cardiovascular disease, nerve damage, kidney damage, and vision loss. However, with proper management, people with diabetes can lead healthy and fulfilling lives.

Diagnosis. Symptoms of Diabetes Type 1 and 2

The diagnosis and symptoms of Type 1 and Type 2 diabetes are different. Here are the details:

Type 1 diabetes:

Diagnosis: Type 1 diabetes is usually diagnosed in childhood or adolescence, but it can also develop in adults. Doctors use blood tests to diagnose Type 1 diabetes by measuring the level of glucose in the blood and testing for antibodies that attack the pancreas.

Symptoms: The symptoms of Type 1 diabetes can develop quickly and include increased thirst and urination, extreme hunger, fatigue, blurred vision, and unexplained weight loss. People with Type 1 diabetes may also experience frequent infections, slow-healing cuts and bruises, and tingling or numbness in the hands and feet.

Type 2 diabetes:

Diagnosis: Type 2 diabetes is often diagnosed later in life, and doctors use blood tests to diagnose the condition. A fasting plasma glucose test or an oral glucose tolerance test may be used to measure the level of glucose in the blood.

Symptoms: The symptoms of Type 2 diabetes can be mild or non-existent in the early stages of the condition, making it difficult to diagnose. Common symptoms include increased thirst and urination, blurry vision, fatigue, slow-healing wounds or infections, and tingling or numbness in the hands and feet. People with Type 2 diabetes may also experience frequent yeast infections or skin infections.

It's important to note that some people with Type 2 diabetes may not experience any symptoms at all, which is why regular screening is recommended for people who are at risk for developing the condition. If you are experiencing any symptoms of diabetes or are concerned about your risk, talk to your doctor about getting screened.

Complications

Both Type 1 and Type 2 diabetes can cause complications if left untreated or poorly managed. Here are some potential complications of diabetes:

- **Cardiovascular disease:** People with diabetes have an increased risk of developing heart disease, stroke, and other cardiovascular problems.
- **Nerve damage:** Over time, high blood sugar levels can damage nerves throughout the body, leading to numbness, tingling, and even loss of sensation in the hands and feet.
- **Kidney damage:** Diabetes can damage the kidneys over time, leading to kidney failure and the need for dialysis or a kidney transplant.
- **Eye damage:** High blood sugar levels can damage the blood vessels in the eyes, leading to diabetic retinopathy, cataracts, and eventually, blindness.
- **Foot problems:** Nerve damage and poor circulation can lead to foot ulcers, infections, and in severe cases, amputation.
- **Skin conditions:** Diabetes can increase the risk of skin infections and other conditions, such as bacterial and fungal infections, itching, and slow-healing wounds.
- **Dental problems:** People with diabetes are more likely to develop gum disease and other dental problems.

These complications can be prevented or minimized by maintaining good blood sugar control through healthy lifestyle habits, medication management, and regular medical checkups.

10 Tips to Control Diabetes

Here are 10 tips that can help people with diabetes manage their condition and maintain good health:

1. **Monitor blood sugar levels regularly:** Check your blood sugar levels regularly and work with your healthcare provider to establish target ranges for fasting and after-meal blood sugar levels.
2. **Follow a healthy eating plan:** Focus on a healthy diet that includes plenty of vegetables, fruits, whole grains, lean protein, and healthy fats. Limit your intake of sugary and processed foods.
3. **Stay physically active:** Exercise regularly to help control blood sugar levels, reduce the risk of heart disease, and maintain a healthy weight.
4. **Take medications as prescribed:** Take your diabetes medications as prescribed by your healthcare provider and follow the recommended dosage and timing.
5. **Manage stress:** Stress can raise blood sugar levels, so it's important to find ways to manage stress, such as meditation, deep breathing, yoga, or counseling.

6. **Maintain a healthy weight:** Achieving and maintaining a healthy weight can help improve blood sugar control and reduce the risk of complications.

7. **Don't smoke:** Smoking increases the risk of heart disease, stroke, and other health problems, so it's important to quit smoking if you smoke.

8. **Get enough sleep:** Getting enough sleep can help improve blood sugar control and overall health. Aim for at least 7-8 hours of sleep per night.

9. **Stay hydrated:** Drink plenty of water and avoid sugary beverages to help maintain good blood sugar control and overall health.

10. **Attend regular medical checkups:** Regular checkups with your healthcare provider can help monitor blood sugar levels, identify potential complications early, and adjust treatment as needed.

What to Eat and What to Avoid

A healthy diet is essential for managing diabetes, and making smart food choices can help keep blood sugar levels in check. Here are some general guidelines on what to eat and what to avoid:

What to Eat:

- **Fruits and vegetables:** These should make up a significant portion of your diet, as they are rich in fiber, vitamins, and minerals.

- **Whole grains:** Whole grains, such as brown rice, quinoa, and whole wheat bread, are rich in fiber and can help regulate blood sugar levels.

- **Lean protein:** Choose lean protein sources, such as chicken, fish, beans, and tofu, to help keep you feeling full and satisfied.

- **Healthy fats:** Foods high in healthy fats, such as nuts, seeds, and avocados, can help improve insulin sensitivity.

What to Avoid:

- **Processed foods:** Processed foods are often high in refined carbohydrates and added sugars, which can lead to blood sugar spikes.

- **Sugary drinks:** Soda, fruit juice, and other sugary drinks can quickly raise blood sugar levels and should be avoided.

- **High-fat and high-sodium foods:** Foods that are high in saturated and trans fats, such as fried foods and fatty meats, can increase the risk of heart disease. Foods high in sodium, such as canned soups and packaged snacks, can lead to high blood pressure.

- **Refined carbohydrates:** Foods made with white flour, such as white bread and pasta, should be limited as they can quickly raise blood sugar levels.

Sugar Alternatives and how to satisfy sugar cravings

For people with diabetes, sugar alternatives can be a helpful tool in managing blood sugar levels. Here are some common sugar alternatives and how they can be used:

- **Stevia:** Stevia is a natural sweetener derived from the leaves of the stevia plant. It has zero calories and does not affect blood sugar levels. It can be used in place of sugar in a variety of recipes and beverages.
- **Erythritol:** Erythritol is a sugar alcohol that is naturally occurring in some fruits and fermented foods. It has zero calories and does not raise blood sugar levels. It can be used in baking and can also be used to sweeten beverages.
- **Xylitol:** Xylitol is another sugar alcohol that has a similar sweetness to sugar but with fewer calories. It does not raise blood sugar levels and can be used in baking and cooking.
- **Monk fruit extract:** Monk fruit extract is a natural sweetener that has zero calories and does not raise blood sugar levels. It can be used in place of sugar in a variety of recipes and beverages.

While sugar alternatives can be a useful tool, it's important to use them in moderation as consuming too much can lead to gastrointestinal issues.

If you're looking to satisfy sugar cravings, there are many ways to do so without consuming refined sugars. Here are some ideas:

- **Fruit:** Fruit is naturally sweet and contains fiber and other beneficial nutrients. Try eating a piece of fruit or adding it to your meals and snacks.
- **Dark chocolate:** Dark chocolate contains antioxidants and can satisfy a sweet tooth. Look for brands that contain at least 70% cocoa solids and enjoy in moderation.
- **Spices:** Spices such as cinnamon and nutmeg can add sweetness to recipes without adding sugar.
- **Nuts and seeds:** Nuts and seeds can provide a satisfying crunch and are a good source of healthy fats and protein.

Treatment for Diabetes: The Importance of Insulin

Insulin is a hormone produced by the pancreas that plays a crucial role in regulating blood sugar levels in the body. For people with diabetes, insulin therapy is often an essential part of their treatment plan.

Type 1 diabetes is a condition in which the body does not produce enough insulin. Insulin therapy is necessary for people with type 1 diabetes to regulate their blood sugar levels. Insulin can be administered via injections or through an insulin pump.

In type 2 diabetes, the body becomes resistant to insulin, and over time, the pancreas may not be able to produce enough insulin to meet the body's needs. In these cases, insulin therapy may also be necessary.

Insulin therapy helps to lower blood sugar levels by allowing glucose to enter the cells of the body where it can be used for energy. When blood sugar levels are too high, it can lead to a range of complications, including damage to the eyes, kidneys, and nerves, as well as an increased risk of heart disease.

Along with insulin therapy, people with diabetes must also follow a healthy lifestyle that includes regular exercise and a balanced diet to help manage their blood sugar levels. It's essential to work closely with a healthcare provider to determine the right insulin regimen and dosage based on individual needs and to monitor blood sugar levels regularly.

How to better understand your glycemic index level?

To better understand your glycemic index level, there are a few things you can do:

1. **Consult with a healthcare professional:** A doctor or a registered dietitian can help you understand your glycemic index level and how it affects your overall health.

2. **Use a blood glucose meter:** A blood glucose meter is a small device that measures the amount of glucose in your blood. Regularly checking your blood glucose levels can give you an idea of how different foods and activities affect your glycemic index level.

3. **Keep a food diary:** Keeping a food diary can help you identify which foods cause your blood sugar levels to spike and which ones don't. This can help you make better choices when it comes to your diet.

4. **Learn about the glycemic index of different foods:** Understanding the glycemic index of different foods can help you make informed decisions about what to eat. High glycemic index foods can cause blood sugar levels to spike quickly, while low glycemic index foods release glucose into the bloodstream more slowly.

5. **Experiment with different foods:** Everyone's body reacts differently to different foods. Experimenting with different foods can help you identify which ones work best for you and which ones to avoid.

Basic Diabetes Ingredient List

If you have diabetes, it's important to have a well-stocked pantry and refrigerator to ensure you have healthy and nutritious ingredients on hand. Here is a basic diabetes ingredient list:

1. **Whole grains:** Whole grains like brown rice, quinoa, whole wheat pasta, and whole grain breads are excellent sources of fiber, vitamins, and minerals.

2. **Fresh fruits and vegetables:** Fresh fruits and vegetables are low in calories and high in fiber, vitamins, and minerals. They can also help you manage your blood sugar levels.

3. **Lean protein:** Lean protein sources like skinless chicken, fish, and tofu can help you build and maintain muscle while keeping you feeling full and satisfied.

4. **Legumes:** Legumes like lentils, chickpeas, and beans are high in fiber and protein, making them an excellent addition to any diabetes-friendly diet.

5. **Nuts and seeds:** Nuts and seeds are rich in healthy fats, protein, and fiber, and they can help you feel full and satisfied.

6. **Low-fat dairy:** Low-fat dairy products like skim milk and low-fat yogurt are excellent sources of calcium and protein.

7. **Healthy fats:** Healthy fats like olive oil, avocado, and nuts can help you maintain healthy cholesterol levels and keep you feeling full and satisfied.

8. **Spices and herbs:** Using spices and herbs like garlic, cinnamon, and ginger can add flavor to your dishes without adding excess salt or sugar.

Remember, the key to managing diabetes is to focus on whole, unprocessed foods and to limit your intake of processed and refined foods that are high in sugar, salt, and unhealthy fats.

Table with different glycemic index products

GLYCEMIC INDEX

LOW   MEDIUM   HIGH

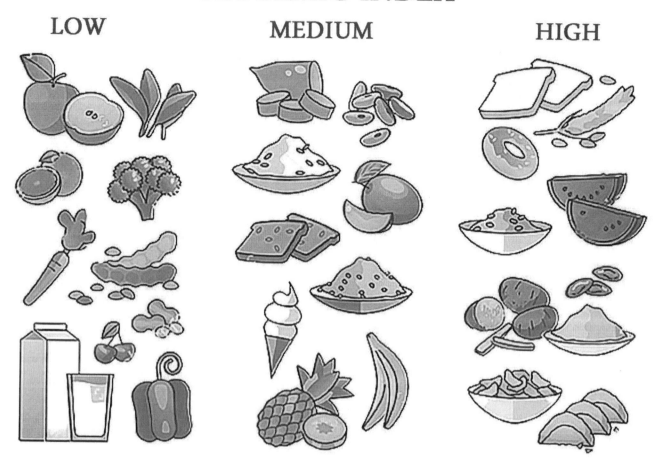

Navigating Labels: A Guide for Diabetic-friendly Products

Understanding food labels is essential for individuals managing diabetes. Here's what you need to know:

1. Sugar Content:

- Check the total sugar content per serving. Look for products labeled "no added sugar" or "sugar-free."
- Avoid products containing high-fructose corn syrup, cane sugar, honey, maple syrup, and other sweeteners.
- Be cautious of terms like "low sugar" or "reduced sugar," as they may still contain significant amounts of sugar.

2. Carbohydrate Content:

- Pay attention to the total carbohydrate content per serving.
- Choose products with lower carbohydrate counts to help manage blood sugar levels.
- Avoid products made with white flour, cornstarch, or other refined carbohydrates.

3. Sodium Levels:

- Keep an eye on the sodium content, especially if you have high blood pressure or are at risk for heart disease.
- Opt for low-sodium or sodium-free versions of products whenever possible.
- Be cautious of sauces like soy sauce, teriyaki sauce, and BBQ sauce, which can be high in sodium.

4. Fat Content:

- Look for products with lower amounts of saturated and trans fats.
- Avoid products containing hydrogenated or partially hydrogenated oils, which indicate the presence of trans fats.
- Choose healthier fats such as olive, avocado, and canola.

5. Artificial Additives and Preservatives:

- Check the ingredient list for artificial preservatives, flavor enhancers, and additives.
- Avoid products containing ingredients like MSG (monosodium glutamate), BHA (butylated hydroxyanisole), BHT (butylated hydroxytoluene), and artificial colors and flavors.
- Choose products with simpler ingredient lists and fewer additives.

6. Hidden Ingredients:

- Be aware of hidden sugars and sweeteners, which may be listed under different names.
- Ingredients like maltose, dextrose, and sucrose can increase blood sugar levels.
- Opt for homemade or sugar-free versions of sauces to avoid hidden sugars.

7. Portion Sizes:

- Pay attention to the serving sizes listed on the nutrition label.
- Adjust portion sizes to avoid consuming excessive sugar, carbohydrates, and sodium.

Products to Be Cautious Of:

Products	Reasons to Be Cautious
Sweetened Beverages	High sugar content, can rapidly raise blood sugar levels
Sugary Snacks	High in carbohydrates and added sugars
Processed Foods	Often contain hidden sugars, unhealthy fats, and high sodium content
Flavored Yogurts	High in added sugars and artificial ingredients
Fruit Juices	Concentrated source of natural sugars

Sauces to Be Cautious Of:

Sauces	Reasons to Be Cautious
BBQ Sauce	Typically high in sugars and may contain additives
Ketchup	Often contains high amounts of added sugars
Teriyaki Sauce	Sweetened with sugars and may contain unhealthy additives
Sweet Chili Sauce	High sugar content, may contain artificial additives
Honey Mustard Sauce	Contains honey, a concentrated source of natural sugars

Ingredients/Preservatives to Be Cautious Of:

Ingredients/Preservatives	Reasons to Be Cautious
High Fructose Corn Syrup	Highly processed sweetener with high sugar content
Artificial Sweeteners	May cause gastrointestinal issues and impact blood sugar levels
Hydrogenated Oils/Trans Fats	Unhealthy fats linked to heart disease and inflammation
MSG (Monosodium Glutamate)	May cause adverse reactions in some individuals
Artificial Flavors and Colors	Often contain chemicals that may have negative health effects

By following these guidelines and being cautious of certain products, sauces, ingredients, and preservatives, individuals with diabetes can make more informed dietary choices to support their health and well-being. Always consult with a healthcare professional or registered dietitian for personalized nutrition advice tailored to your specific needs.

Substitution Guide for Diabetics

Making smart food choices is essential for managing diabetes. Here's a detailed guide to common foods and their healthier alternatives that can be used in air fryer recipes:

Common Foods	Alternative/ Substitute	Reasons to Substitute
White Rice	Brown Rice	Brown rice has a lower glycemic index and higher fiber content, which helps regulate blood sugar levels better.
White Bread	Whole Grain Bread	Whole grain bread contains more fiber and nutrients than white bread, leading to slower digestion and better blood sugar control.
Potatoes	Sweet Potatoes	Sweet potatoes have a lower glycemic index and are rich in fiber, vitamins, and minerals, making them a healthier option for managing blood sugar.
Regular Pasta	Whole Wheat Pasta	Whole wheat pasta is higher in fiber and nutrients compared to regular pasta, providing more sustained energy and better blood sugar management.
Sugary Cereals	Oatmeal	Oatmeal is a high-fiber, low-glycemic index option that provides long-lasting energy and helps stabilize blood sugar levels.
Fried Foods	Air-Fried Foods	Air-frying reduces the amount of unhealthy fats and calories in fried foods, making them a healthier choice for individuals with diabetes.
Sugary Beverages	Infused Water or Herbal Tea	Infused water or herbal tea provides hydration without the added sugars and calories found in sugary beverages, helping to manage blood sugar levels.
Processed Meats	Lean Protein Sources (e.g., Chicken Breast, Fish)	Lean protein sources are lower in saturated fats and healthier for the heart, contributing to better overall health and blood sugar management.
High-Sugar Sauces	Homemade Sauces with Natural Sweeteners	Homemade sauces made with natural sweeteners like stevia or erythritol offer flavor without the negative impact on blood sugar levels associated with high-sugar sauces.
Candy and Sweets	Fresh Fruit	Fresh fruit provides natural sweetness along with vitamins, minerals, and fiber, making it a healthier alternative to candy and sweets for managing blood sugar levels.

Chapter 1. Breakfast and Eggs

Air Fryer Breakfast Egg Rolls

Serving: 4 | Preparation time: 10 minutes | Cooking Time: 10 minutes.

Ingredients:

• 4 large eggs
• 1 oz (30g) chopped onion
• 1 oz (30g) chopped mushrooms
• 4 egg roll wrappers
• 1 oz (30g) chopped bell pepper
• 1 tbsp olive oil, salt

Instructions:

1. Preheat the air fryer to 400°F (205°C).
2. In a bowl, beat the eggs and add the chopped onion, salt bell pepper, and mushrooms.
3. Brush olive oil onto one side of each egg roll wrapper.
4. Add about 1/4 cup of the egg mixture onto the center of each wrapper.
5. Roll up the wrapper tightly, tucking in the sides as you go.
6. Place the egg rolls in the air fryer basket, seam side down, and cook for 10-12 minutes until golden brown and crispy.
7. Serve hot and enjoy!

Nutritional values:

Calories: 225kcal | Fat: 13g | Protein: 12g | Carbs: 16g | Net carbs: 12g | Fiber: 4g | Cholesterol: 220mg | Sodium: 316mg | Potassium: 202mg

Air Fryer Breakfast Casserole

Serving: 4 | Preparation Time: 25 minutes

Ingredients:

• 6 large eggs
• 4 oz (120ml) milk
• 4 slices bacon, cooked and crumbled
• 1.88 oz (50g) shredded cheddar cheese
• 0.88 oz (25g) diced bell peppers
• 0.88 oz (25 g) diced onion
• Salt and pepper to taste
• Cooking spray

Instructions:

1. Preheat the air fryer to 350°F (175°C).
2. In a bowl, whisk together eggs, milk, salt, and pepper.
3. Spray a baking dish or a small oven-safe dish that fits in your air fryer with cooking spray.
4. Spread the cooked and crumbled bacon, diced bell peppers, and diced onion evenly in the baking dish.
5. Pour the egg mixture over the ingredients in the baking dish.
6. Sprinkle shredded cheddar cheese on top.
7. Place the baking dish in the air fryer basket and cook for 15-20 minutes or until the eggs are set and the top is golden brown.
8. Remove from the air fryer and let it cool slightly before serving.

Note: use almond milk for dairy-free option, use dairy-free cheese for dairy-free option.

Nutritional values:

Calories: 248kcal | Fat: 18g | Protein: 17g | Carbs: 2g | Net carbs: 2g | Fiber: 0g | Cholesterol: 305mg | Sodium: 338mg | Potassium: 191mg

Air Fryer Breakfast Burritos

Serving: 4 | Preparation time: 10 minutes | Cooking time: 8-10 minutes

Ingredients:

• 4 low-carb tortillas
• 4 large eggs
• 1 oz (25g) shredded cheddar cheese
• 2 oz (60ml) unsweetened almond milk
• 2 slices of bacon, cooked and crumbled
• 0.3 oz (10g) chopped green onions
• Salt and pepper to taste

Instructions:

1. In a medium-sized mixing bowl, whisk together the eggs, almond milk, salt, and pepper.
2. Preheat the air fryer to 375°F (190°C).
3. Place the tortillas on a flat surface and divide the egg mixture among them.
4. Top each tortilla with shredded cheese, crumbled bacon, and chopped green onions.
5. Roll up the tortillas tightly and place them seam-side down in the air fryer basket.
6. Air fry for 8-10 minutes or until the burritos are golden brown and crispy.
7. Serve immediately and enjoy!

Nutritional values:

Calories: 250kcal | Fat: 16g | Protein: 16g | Carbs: 13g | Net carbs: 7g | Fiber: 6g | Cholesterol: 210mg | Sodium: 460mg | Potassium: 180mg

Air Fryer Vegetable Frittata

Servings: 4 | Preparation time: 10-15 minutes | Cooking time: 10-12 minutes

Ingredients:

• 6 large eggs
• 1 oz (30g) red bell pepper, chopped
• 1 oz (30g) onion, chopped
• 1 oz (30g) shredded cheddar cheese
• 0.5 oz (15g) green bell pepper, chopped
• 2 oz (60ml) milk
• Salt and pepper to taste
• Cooking spray

Instructions:

1. Preheat the air fryer to 350°F (180°C).
2. In a bowl, whisk together the eggs, milk, salt, and pepper.
3. Add the chopped bell peppers and onions to the bowl and stir to combine.
4. Grease a 6-inch (15 cm) baking dish that fits in the air fryer basket with cooking spray.
5. Pour the egg mixture into the baking dish.
6. Sprinkle the shredded cheddar cheese over the top of the egg mixture.
7. Place the baking dish in the air fryer basket and cook for 15-18 minutes, or until the frittata is set and the cheese is melted and golden brown.
8. Remove the baking dish from the air fryer and let cool for a few minutes before slicing and serving.

Nutritional values:

Calories: 230kcal | Fat: 16g | Protein: 16g | Carbs: 5g | Net carbs: 3g | Fiber: 2g | Cholesterol: 415mg | Sodium: 390mg | Potassium: 280mg.

Air Fryer Sweet Potato Hash Browns

Serving: 4 | Preparation time: 10 minutes | Cooking time: 15 minutes

Ingredients:

• 17.64 oz (500g) sweet potatoes, peeled and grated
• 1/2 tsp salt
• 1 oz (30g) almond flour
• 1 tsp smoked paprika
• 1 tsp garlic powder
• 2 tbsp avocado oil

Instructions:

1. Preheat the air fryer to 380°F (193°C).
2. In a large mixing bowl, combine grated sweet potatoes, almond flour, smoked paprika, garlic powder, and salt. Mix until well combined.
3. Drizzle avocado oil over the sweet potato mixture and mix well.
4. Form the mixture into small patties, about 2-3 inches in diameter.
5. Place the sweet potato patties into the air fryer basket, leaving some space between each patty.
6. Cook the hash browns for 8-10 minutes, flipping them halfway through.
7. Once the hash browns are crispy and golden brown, remove them from the air fryer and serve hot.

Nutritional values:

Calories: 175kcal | Fat: 10g | Protein: 3g | Carbs: 19g | Net carbs: 14g | Fiber: 5g | Cholesterol: 0mg | Sodium: 247mg | Potassium: 320mg

Air Fryer Egg Muffins

Serving: 6 egg muffins | Preparation time: 15 minutes | Cooking time: 10-12 minutes

Ingredients:

- 6 eggs
- 2 oz (60 ml) unsweetened almond milk
- 0.88 oz (25g) chopped spinach
- 0.88 oz (25g) chopped red bell pepper
- 0.88 oz (25g) chopped onion
- 0.88 oz (25g) sliced mushrooms
- Salt and pepper, to taste
- Cooking spray

Instructions:

1. Preheat the air fryer to 300°F (150°C).
2. In a mixing bowl, beat the eggs, salt, pepper, and almond milk together.
3. Add the chopped spinach, red bell pepper, onion, and mushrooms to the egg mixture. Stir to combine.
4. Grease a muffin tin with cooking spray.
5. Pour the egg mixture evenly into the muffin tin.
6. Place the muffin tin in the air fryer basket and cook for 10-12 minutes, or until the eggs are set and cooked through.
7. Remove the muffin tin from the air fryer and let the egg muffins cool for a few minutes before removing them from the muffin tin.
8. Serve and enjoy!

Nutritional values:

Calories: 83 kcal | Fat: 6g | Protein: 6g | Carbs: 2g | Net carbs: 1g | Fiber: 1g | Cholesterol: 164mg | Sodium: 101mg | Potassium:96mg

Air Fryer Avocado Egg Boats

Serving: 4 | Preparation time: 10 Minutes | Cooking Time: 10 minutes

Ingredients:

- 2 ripe avocados
- 4 large eggs
- 2 tbsp chopped fresh cilantro
- 1/2 tsp chili powder
- ¼ tsp ground cumin
- Salt and pepper to taste

Instructions:

1. Preheat the air fryer to 375°F (190°C).
2. Cut the avocados in half lengthwise and remove the pits.

3. Scoop out a little bit of flesh from the center of each avocado half to make room for the egg.
4. Crack one egg into each avocado half.
5. Sprinkle each avocado half with cilantro, chili powder, cumin, salt, and pepper.
6. Place the avocado halves in the air fryer basket.
7. Cook for 12-15 minutes or until the egg whites are set and the yolks are cooked to your liking.
8. Serve immediately.

Nutritional values:

Calories: 231kcal | Fat: 20g | Protein: 8g | Carbs: 9g | Net carbs: 3g | Fiber: 6g | Cholesterol: 186mg | Sodium: 75mg | Potassium: 599mg

Air Fryer Ham and Cheese Omelette

Servings: 2 | Preparation time: 5 minutes | Cooking time: 8 minutes

Ingredients:

- 3 eggs
- 0.88 oz (25g) shredded cheddar cheese
- 0.88 oz (25g) diced ham
- 1/4 tsp salt
- 1/4 tsp black pepper
- 1 tsp olive oil

Instructions:

1. Preheat the air fryer to 350°F (180°C).
2. In a bowl, beat the eggs and add the shredded cheese, diced ham, salt, and black pepper. Mix well.
3. Grease a small heat-proof dish or ramekin with olive oil. Pour the egg mixture into the dish.
4. Place the dish in the air fryer basket and cook for 10-12 minutes, or until the eggs are set and the cheese is melted and bubbly.
5. Carefully remove the dish from the air fryer basket and let it cool for a few minutes.
6. Serve the omelette hot with your favorite breakfast sides.

Nutritional values:

Calories: 290kcal | Fat: 22g | Protein: 19g | Carbs: 2g | Net carbs: 2g | Fiber: 0g | Cholesterol: 416mg | Sodium: 820mg | Potassium: 216mg.

Air Fryer Cinnamon French Toast Sticks

Servings: 2 | Preparation time: 10 minutes | Cooking time: 5-6 minutes

Ingredients:

• 4 oz (120g) slices of low-carb bread, cut into strips
• 2 eggs
• 2 oz (60ml) milk
• 1 tsp ground cinnamon
• 1 tsp vanilla extract
• 2 tbsp unsalted butter, melted
• Maple syrup, for serving

Instructions:

1. Preheat the air fryer to 370°F (187°C).
2. In a shallow dish, whisk together the eggs, milk, cinnamon, and vanilla extract.
3. Dip the bread strips into the egg mixture, making sure to coat both sides.
4. Brush the air fryer basket with melted butter and arrange the bread strips in a single layer.
5. Cook in the air fryer for 5-6 minutes, flipping halfway through, until golden brown and crispy.
6. Serve with maple syrup.

Note: The use of too much maple syrup might affect your sugar level, be careful of excess sugar or honey

Nutritional values:

Calories: 294kcal | Fat: 14g | Protein: 10g | Carbs: 32g | Net carbs: 29g | Fiber: 3g | Cholesterol: 190mg | Sodium: 418mg | Potassium: 163mg

Air Fryer Oatmeal Raisin Breakfast Bars

Servings: 8 bars | Preparation time: 10 minutes | Cooking time: 15-20 minutes

Ingredients:

• 5.3 oz (160g) old-fashioned rolled oats
• 2 oz (60g) raisins
• 1 oz (30g) almond flour
• 2 oz (60ml) unsweetened applesauce
• 1 oz (30ml) maple syrup
• 2 oz (60ml) almond milk
• 1 tsp ground cinnamon
• Pinch of salt

Instructions:

1. Preheat the air fryer to 370°F (187°C).
2. In a large bowl, combine the oats, raisins, almond flour, cinnamon, and salt.
3. In a separate bowl, whisk together the applesauce, maple syrup, and almond milk.
4. Add the wet ingredients to the dry ingredients and mix well.
5. Line an 8x8 inch (20x20 cm) baking dish with parchment paper and transfer the mixture to the dish.
6. Use a spatula to press the mixture down firmly and evenly.
7. Place the baking dish in the air fryer and cook at 320°F (160°C) for 15-20 minutes, or until golden brown on top.
8. Remove from the air fryer and let cool completely before slicing into bars.
9. Serve and enjoy!

Nutritional values:

Calories: 150kcal | Fat: 4.2g | Protein: 4.2g | Carbs: 26.4g | Net carbs: 18.4g | Fiber: 8 g | Cholesterol: 0mg | Sodium: 15mg | Potassium: 220mg

Air Fryer Blueberry Muffins

Serving: 4 | Preparation Time: 25 minutes

Ingredients:

• 6 oz (180 g) almond flour
• 1 oz (30 g) coconut flour
• 1/2 tsp baking powder
• 1/4 tsp baking soda
• 1/4 tsp salt
• 2 oz (60ml) coconut oil, melted
• 2 oz (60ml) unsweetened almond milk
• 1 oz (30 ml) maple syrup
• 2 large eggs
• 1 tsp vanilla extracts
• 5 oz (150g) fresh blueberries

Instructions:

1. Preheat the air fryer to 350°F (175°C).
2. In a large bowl, whisk together almond flour, coconut flour, baking powder, baking soda, and salt.

3. In a separate bowl, whisk together melted coconut oil, almond milk, maple syrup, eggs, and vanilla extract.

4. Add the wet ingredients to the dry ingredients and stir until well combined.

5. Gently fold in the fresh blueberries.

6. Line a muffin tin with paper liners or use silicone muffin cups. Fill each cup with the muffin batter, about 3/4 full.

7. Place the muffin tin in the air fryer basket. If your air fryer is small, you may need to cook the muffins in batches.

8. Air fry for 12-15 minutes or until a toothpick inserted into the center of a muffin comes out clean.

9. Remove the muffins from the air fryer and let them cool for a few minutes before serving.

Note: The use of too much sugar or honey might affect your sugar level, be careful of excess sugar or honey

Nutritional values:

Calories: 195kcal | Fat: 16g | Protein: 6g | Carbs: 9g | Net carbs: 6g | Fiber: 3g | Cholesterol: 37mg | Sodium: 162mg | Potassium: 94mg

Air Fryer Breakfast Quesadillas

Serving: 1 quesadilla | Prep time: 10 minutes | Cook time: 5-6 minutes

Ingredients:

• 2 large eggs
• 2 small low-carb tortillas
• 2 tbsp of diced green chilies
• 1 oz (30g) shredded cheddar cheese
• 1 oz (30g) cooked and crumbled breakfast sausage
• Salt and pepper to taste

Instructions:

1. Preheat the air fryer to 350°F (175°C).

2. In a small bowl, whisk the eggs with salt and pepper.

3. Place one tortilla on a flat surface and sprinkle with half of the cheese, sausage, and green chilies. Pour half of the egg mixture on top.

4. Top with the other tortilla and press gently.

5. Transfer the quesadilla to the air fryer basket and cook for 5-6 minutes or until golden and crispy.

6. Remove from the air fryer and let it cool for a minute before slicing and serving.

Nutritional values:

Calories: 303kcal | Fat: 19g | Protein: 17g | Carbs: 16g | Net carbs: 14g | Fiber: 2g | Cholesterol: 253mg | Sodium: 608mg | Potassium: 167mg

Air Fryer Spinach and Feta Breakfast Pockets

Serving: 4 pockets | Preparation time: 20 minutes.

Ingredients:

• 1 sheet of filo pastry, thawed
• 2 eggs, lightly beaten
• 2.5 oz (75g) crumbled feta cheese
• 1 oz (30g) chopped spinach
• 1/4 tsp garlic powder
• Salt and pepper, to taste
• Cooking spray

Instructions:

1. Preheat the air fryer to 375°F (190°C).

2. In a bowl, mix together the beaten eggs, crumbled feta cheese, chopped spinach, garlic powder, salt, and pepper.

3. Roll out the puff pastry sheet and cut into 4 equal squares.

4. Spoon the egg mixture onto one half of each square, leaving a small border around the edge.

5. Fold the other half of the puff pastry over the egg mixture and use a fork to crimp the edges closed.

6. Spray the air fryer basket with cooking spray.

7. Place the breakfast pockets in the air fryer basket, making sure they are not touching each other.

8. Air fry for 8-10 minutes or until the pastry is golden brown and the egg is cooked through.

9. Serve hot.

Nutritional values:

Calories: 320kcal | Fat: 22g | Protein: 10g | Carbs: 21g | Net carbs: 20g | Fiber: 1g | Cholesterol: 130mg | Sodium: 500mg | Potassium: 160mg

Air Fryer Breakfast Flatbread

Serving: 4 | Preparation Time: 10 minutes | Cook Time: 10 minutes

Ingredients:

- 4 oz (120g) low-carb bread
- 4 large eggs
- 2 oz (60g) shredded cheddar cheese
- Salt and pepper to taste
- Optional toppings: diced tomatoes, chopped green onions, hot sauce
- Cooking spray

Instructions:

1. Preheat the air fryer to 350°F (175°C).
2. Lightly spray or brush the low-carb bread with cooking spray or oil on both sides.
3. Place the low-carb bread in the air fryer basket in a single layer.
4. Cook in the air fryer at 350°F (175°C) for 2-3 minutes to lightly toast the flatbreads.
5. Remove the low-carb bread from the air fryer and set them aside.
6. Crack one egg onto each low-carb bread, ensuring it is spread evenly.
7. Sprinkle the shredded cheddar cheese, and chopped fresh herbs evenly over the eggs.
8. Season with salt and pepper to taste.
9. Return the topped low-carb bread to the air fryer basket.
10. Cook in the air fryer at 350°F (175°C) for 8-10 minutes, or until the eggs are cooked to your desired doneness and the cheese has melted.
11. Carefully remove the breakfast flatbreads from the air fryer and let them cool slightly before serving.
12. Slice into wedges or squares and serve as a delicious breakfast or brunch option.
13. Enjoy your tasty Air Fryer Breakfast Flatbread!

Note: You can customize the toppings based on your preferences by adding vegetables, herbs, or other ingredients you enjoy in your breakfast dishes.

Nutritional values:

260kcal | Fat: 15g | Protein: 16g | Carbohydrates: 16g | Fiber: 1g | Cholesterol: 215mg | Sodium: 420mg | Potassium: 120mg

Air Fryer Bacon and Egg Cups

Serving: 4 cups | Prep time: 10 minutes | Cook time: 15 minutes

Ingredients:

- 6 slices bacon
- 4 large eggs
- 1 oz (30g) shredded cheddar
- Fresh chives, chopped, for garnish
- Salt and pepper, to taste
- Cooking spray

Instructions:

1. Preheat the air fryer to 350°F (180°C).
2. Grease 4 cups of a muffin tin with non-stick cooking spray.
3. Cook bacon in the air fryer for 5-7 minutes, or until crispy. Remove from the air fryer and let cool.
4. Once cool, chop the bacon into small pieces.
5. Crack one egg into each muffin cup.
6. Add chopped bacon to each cup.
7. Sprinkle shredded cheese over the bacon and egg mixture.
8. Season with salt and pepper.
9. Place the muffin tin in the air fryer and cook for 8-10 minutes or until the egg is set.
10. Remove from the air fryer and let cool for a few minutes.
11. Garnish with fresh chives and serve.

Nutritional values:

Calories: 228kcal | Fat: 18g | Protein: 14g | Carbs: 1g | Fiber: 0g | Cholesterol: 235mg | Sodium: 405mg | Potassium: 155mg

Air Fryer Baked Eggs in Tomato Sauce

Serving: 4 Preparation Time: 10 Minutes

Ingredients:

- 2 eggs
- 4 oz (120ml) tomato sauce
- 0.88 oz (25g) grated Parmesan cheese
- 1 tbsp chopped fresh parsley
- Salt and black pepper, to taste
- 1 tbsp olive oil

Instructions:

1. Preheat the air fryer to 375°F (190°C).
2. In a small bowl, mix together the tomato sauce, grated Parmesan cheese, chopped parsley, salt, and black pepper.
3. Drizzle olive oil on the bottom of a small oven-safe ramekin or dish.
4. Spoon the tomato sauce mixture into the bottom of the ramekin or dish.
5. Crack the eggs into the ramekin or dish, on top of the tomato sauce mixture.
6. Place the ramekin or dish into the air fryer basket and cook for 6-8 minutes, or until the egg whites are set and the yolks are cooked to your desired consistency.
7. Remove the ramekin or dish from the air fryer using oven mitts and allow to cool for a few minutes before serving.
8. Serve hot with toast or crusty bread.

Nutritional values:

Calories: 225kcal | Fat: 16g | Protein: 12g | Carbs: 7g | Net carbs: 5g | Fiber: 2g | Cholesterol: 328mg | Sodium: 657mg | Potassium: 371mg.

Air Fryer Breakfast Sausage

Serving: 4 | Preparation Time: 10 Minutes

Ingredients:

- 15.2 oz (454g) ground pork
- 1 tsp maple syrup
- 1 tsp salt
- 1/2 tsp ground black pepper
- 1/2 tsp dried sage
- 1/2 tsp dried thyme
- 1/4 tsp garlic powder
- 1/4 tsp onion powder

Instructions:

1. Preheat the air fryer to 360°F (182°C).
2. In a large bowl, mix together ground pork, maple syrup, salt, black pepper, sage, thyme, garlic powder, and onion powder.
3. Divide the mixture into 8 equal parts and form into patties.
4. Place the patties in the air fryer basket in a single layer.

5. Cook for 8-10 minutes, flipping once halfway through cooking time, until fully cooked.
6. Serve hot and enjoy!

Note: The use of too much maple syrup might affect your sugar level, be careful of excess sugar or honey

Nutritional values:

Calories: 220kcal | Fat: 17g | Protein: 13g | Carbs: 3g | Net carbs: 2g | Fiber: 1 g | Cholesterol: 60mg | Sodium: 330mg | Potassium: 234mg

Air Fryer Breakfast Stuffed Peppers

Serving: 4 | Prep time: 10 minutes | Cook time: 15 minutes

Ingredients:

- 4 bell peppers, halved and seeded
- 6 large eggs
- 2 oz (60ml) milk
- 1.9 oz (56g) shredded cheddar cheese
- 1.4 oz (40g) diced onion
- 1.4 oz (40g) diced tomato
- Salt and pepper, to taste
- Cooking spray

Instructions:

1. Preheat your air fryer to 350°F (180°C).
2. In a mixing bowl, beat together eggs, milk, salt, and pepper.
3. Add in diced onions and tomatoes, and mix well.
4. Spray the inside of each pepper half with cooking spray and fill with egg mixture.
5. Sprinkle shredded cheddar cheese on top of the egg mixture.
6. Place the stuffed peppers in the air fryer basket and cook for 10-12 minutes or until the eggs are set and the cheese is melted.
7. Serve hot.

Nutritional values:

Calories: 157kcal | Fat: 9g | Protein: 12g | Carbs: 8g | Net carbs: 6g | Fiber: 2g | Cholesterol: 223mg | Sodium: 171mg | Potassium: 318mg

Air Fryer Sausage and Egg Breakfast Sandwich

Serving: 4 | Preparation Time: 10 Minutes | Cooking Time: 10 Minutes

Ingredients:

- 16 oz (454g) low-carb muffins
- 16 oz (454g) sausage patties
- 6 large eggs
- 4 oz (113g) slices of cheese
- Salt and pepper to taste

Instructions:

1. Preheat the air fryer to 375°F (190°C).
2. Cook the sausage patties in the air fryer for 5-7 minutes, or until browned and fully cooked.
3. While the sausage patties are cooking, crack an egg into each compartment of an egg bite mold, season with salt and pepper, and whisk with a fork.
4. Place the egg bite mold into the air fryer and cook for 6-8 minutes, or until the eggs are set.
5. Once the sausage patties and eggs are done cooking, toast the muffins in the air fryer for 1-2 minutes.
6. Assemble the breakfast sandwiches by placing a sausage patty, a slice of cheese, and a cooked egg onto each muffin.
7. Serve immediately and enjoy!

Nutritional value:

Calories: 440 kcal | Fat: 26 g | Protein: 27 g | Carbohydrates: 24 g | Fiber: 2 g | Sugar: 2 g | Sodium: 840 mg

Air Fryer Hash Brown Egg Nests

Serving: 4 | Preparation time: 15 minutes

Ingredients:

- 16.82 oz (500g) frozen hash browns, thawed
- 2 tbsp olive oil
- 1/2 tsp salt
- 1/4 tsp black pepper
- 4 large eggs
- 1 oz (28g) shredded cheddar cheese
- 0.6 oz (15g) green onion, thinly sliced
- Cooking spray

Instructions:

1. Preheat the air fryer to 375°F (190°C).
2. In a large mixing bowl, combine the hash browns, olive oil, salt, and black pepper. Mix well.
3. Grease four ramekins with cooking spray.
4. Divide the hash brown mixture into four portions and press each portion into the prepared ramekins, forming nests.
5. Crack an egg into each nest and sprinkle with shredded cheddar cheese.
6. Place the ramekins in the air fryer basket and cook for 12-15 minutes or until the eggs are cooked to your liking.
7. Garnish with sliced green onions and serve hot.

Nutritional values:

Calories: 287kcal | Fat: 19g | Protein: 10g | Carbs: 20g | Net carbs: 17g | Fiber: 3g | Cholesterol: 193mg | Sodium: 510mg | Potassium: 446mg

Air Fryer Mini Frittatas

Serving: 3-4 people (makes 6 frittatas) | Preparation time: 10 minutes

Ingredients:

- 6 large eggs
- 2 oz (60ml) milk
- 0.88 oz (28g) shredded cheese
- 1 oz (30g) diced bell peppers
- 1.2 oz (35g) of diced ham
- Cooking spray
- Salt and pepper to taste

Instructions:

1. Preheat your air fryer to 350°F (175°C).
2. In a medium mixing bowl, whisk together the eggs, milk, salt, and pepper.
3. Add the shredded cheese, diced bell peppers, and diced ham to the mixing bowl, and stir everything together.
4. Spray the wells of a muffin tin with cooking spray, then pour the egg mixture into the wells until they are about 3/4 full.
5. Place the muffin tin in the air fryer and cook for 8-10 minutes, or until the frittatas are fully cooked and slightly browned on top.

6. Remove the muffin tin from the air fryer and let the frittatas cool for a few minutes before removing them from the tin.

7. Serve and enjoy!

Nutritional values:
Calories: 110kcal | Fat: 7g | Protein: 9g | Carbs: 2g | Net carbs: 2g | Fiber: 0g | Cholesterol: 193mg | Sodium: 182mg | Potassium: 102mg

Air Fryer Breakfast Taquitos

Serving: 4 | Preparation time: 15 minutes | Cooking time: 12 minutes

Ingredients:
• 11.3 oz (320g) small low carb tortillas
• 6 large eggs
• 2 oz (60ml) milk
• 2 oz (56g) shredded cheddar cheese
• 2 oz (56g) cooked breakfast sausage, crumbled
• 1 oz (30g) diced green bell pepper
• 1 oz (30g) diced red onion
• Salt and pepper, to taste
• Cooking spray

Instructions:
1. Preheat your air fryer to 400°F (200°C).

2. In a mixing bowl, whisk together the eggs and milk until fully combined. Stir in the shredded cheese, crumbled breakfast sausage, diced green bell pepper, and diced red onion. Season with salt and pepper to taste.

3. Place a tortilla on a flat surface and spoon some of the egg mixture onto the center of the tortilla. Roll up tightly into a taquito shape and place seam-side down on a plate. Repeat with the remaining tortillas and egg mixture.

4. Spray the air fryer basket with cooking spray. Place the taquitos in the air fryer basket, making sure they are not touching each other.

5. Cook the taquitos for 6-8 minutes, flipping them over halfway through the cooking time, or until golden brown and crispy.

6. Serve immediately with your favorite breakfast condiments, such as salsa, sour cream, or guacamole.

Nutritional values:
Calories: 236kcal | Fat: 13g | Protein: 12g | Carbs: 18g | Net carbs: 16g | Fiber: 2g | Cholesterol: 171mg | Sodium: 416mg | Potassium: 145mg

Air Fryer Turkey Sausage and Egg Breakfast Pockets

Serving: 4 | Preparation time: 10 minutes

Ingredients:
• 4 small low carb tortillas (6-inch diameter)
• 4 large eggs
• 2 oz (60g) shredded cheddar cheese
• 5.20 oz (170g) turkey sausage links
• 1 oz (30ml) milk
• 1 oz (30g) chopped green onion
• 1 oz (30g) chopped pepper
• Salt and pepper, to taste
• Cooking spray or oil

For serving (optional):
• Salsa
• Avocado slices
• Sour cream

Instructions:
1. Preheat the air fryer to 375°F (190°C).

2. Spray the air fryer basket with cooking spray.

3. In a large bowl, whisk together the eggs, milk, chopped peppers, and onion. Add salt and pepper to taste.

4. Pour the egg mixture into the air fryer basket and cook for 5-7 minutes or until the eggs are set.

5. Meanwhile, cook the turkey sausages in a skillet until browned and cooked through.

6. Cut the pita pockets in half and stuff each pocket with equal amounts of cooked eggs, sausage slices, and shredded cheese.

7. Place the stuffed pita pockets in the air fryer basket and cook for 4-5 minutes or until the cheese is melted and the pockets are crispy.

8. Serve hot with optional toppings such as salsa, avocado slices, and sour cream.

Nutritional values:
Calories: 383kcal | Fat: 17g | Protein: 23g | Carbs: 35g | Net carbs: 31g | Fiber: 4g | Cholesterol: 247mg | Sodium: 812mg | Potassium: 395mg

Air Fryer Breakfast Tostadas

Servings: 4 | Preparation Time: 10 Minutes

Ingredients:

- 4 low-carb tortillas
- 4 eggs
- 5 oz (75g) black beans, drained and rinsed
- 2.5 oz (75g) shredded cheddar cheese
- 4.1 oz (125ml) salsa
- 1 avocado, diced
- Salt and pepper to taste
- Cooking spray

Instructions:

1. Preheat your air fryer to 400°F (200°C).
2. Lightly coat each tortilla with cooking spray on both sides.
3. Place the tortillas in the air fryer basket, making sure they don't overlap, and air fry for 4-5 minutes, until they become crispy and golden brown.
4. In a skillet, scramble the eggs and season with salt and pepper to taste.
5. Assemble the tostadas by topping each tortilla with scrambled eggs, black beans, sliced avocado, shredded cheddar cheese, and salsa.
6. Return the tostadas to the air fryer basket and air fry for an additional 2-3 minutes, until the cheese has melted.
7. Serve hot and enjoy!

Nutritional values:

Calories: 371kcal | Fat: 20g | Protein: 24g | Carbs: 27g | Net carbs: 20g | Fiber: 7g | Sugar: 2g | Sodium: 391mg | Potassium: 589mg

Air Fryer Ham and Cheese Breakfast Pockets

Serving: 4 | Preparation time: 15 minutes

Ingredients:

- 8 oz (240g) refrigerated filo pastry
- 3.88 oz (113g) slices deli ham
- 1.88 oz (56.7g) shredded cheddar cheese
- Salt and pepper to taste
- Cooking spray
- 2 eggs, scrambled

Instructions:

1. Preheat your air fryer to 375°F (190°C).
2. Unroll the filo pastry and separate into 4 rectangles.
3. Place one slice of ham on each rectangle of filo pastry.
4. In a small bowl, mix the scrambled eggs, shredded cheese, salt, and pepper.
5. Spoon the egg and cheese mixture evenly over the ham.
6. Fold the filo pastry over to form a pocket and seal the edges by pressing down with a fork.
7. Spray the air fryer basket with cooking spray.
8. Place the pockets in the air fryer basket and cook for 10-12 minutes or until golden brown.
9. Serve hot and enjoy your Air Fryer Ham and Cheese Breakfast Pockets!

Nutritional value:

Calories: 300kcal | Fat: 19g | Protein: 14g | Carbs: 17g | Net carbs: 16g | Fiber: 1g | Cholesterol: 129mg | Sodium: 834mg | Potassium: 120mg

Air Fryer Breakfast Empanadas

Serving: 4 | Preparation time: 20 minutes

Ingredients:

- 11.3 oz (320g) 1 sheet filo pastry, thawed
- 6 large eggs
- 2 tbsp milk
- 1/2 tsp salt
- 1/4 tsp black pepper
- 1/4 tsp garlic powder
- 1/4 tsp onion powder
- 1.88 oz (56g) shredded cheddar cheese
- 2.04 oz (64g) cooked breakfast sausage, crumbled
- 1 oz (30g) diced green onions
- 1 egg, beaten (for egg wash)
- Cooking spray

Instructions

1. Preheat the air fryer to 375°F (190°C).
2. In a medium bowl, whisk together the eggs, milk, salt, pepper, garlic powder, and onion powder.

3. Lightly grease the air fryer basket or tray to prevent sticking.

4. Pour the whisked egg mixture into the preheated and greased air fryer basket or tray.

5. Cook the scrambled eggs in the air fryer for about 3-4 minutes, stirring occasionally, until they are just set and no longer runny.

6. Once the scrambled eggs are cooked, remove them from the air fryer and set them aside.

7. Now, let's continue with the remaining steps to make the empanadas:

8. On a lightly floured surface, roll out the filo pastry to 1/4-inch thickness. Cut the pastry into 4 equal squares.

9. On each square, add a spoonful of the previously cooked scrambled eggs, followed by some shredded cheese, crumbled breakfast sausage, and diced green onions.

10. Fold the pastry over to create a triangle and press the edges together to seal.

11. Use a fork to crimp the edges and create a decorative pattern.

12. Brush the empanadas with egg wash.

13. Place the empanadas in the air fryer basket and cook for 10-12 minutes or until they turn golden brown and crispy.

14. Serve the delicious and flavorful scrambled eggs empanadas hot, and enjoy a delightful meal!

Nutritional values:
Calories: 379kcal | Fat: 28g | Protein: 15g | Carbs: 16g | Net carbs: 15g | Fiber: 1g | Cholesterol: 236mg | Sodium: 615mg | Potassium: 149mg.

Air Fryer Breakfast Tacos

Serving: 4 | Preparation time: 10 minutes

Ingredients:

• 4 oz (120g) low-carb tortillas
• 4 eggs
• 2 oz (60ml) milk
• 1.88 oz (56g) shredded cheddar cheese
• 2.30 oz (70g) avocado, sliced
• 1.50 oz (40g) chopped fresh cilantro
• Salt and pepper to taste
• Cooking spray

• Optional toppings: salsa, diced tomatoes, jalapeños

Instructions:

1. Preheat your air fryer to 350°F (175°C).

2. In a small bowl, whisk together the eggs and milk. Season with salt and pepper to taste.

3. Spray the air fryer basket with cooking spray.

4. Place the tortillas in the air fryer basket and cook for 1-2 minutes until they are slightly crispy.

5. Remove the tortillas from the air fryer and divide the egg mixture evenly among them.

6. Top each tortilla with shredded cheese.

7. Place the tortillas back in the air fryer and cook for 4-5 minutes until the eggs are set and the cheese is melted.

8. Remove the tacos from the air fryer and top with sliced avocado and fresh cilantro. Serve with your favorite toppings.

Nutritional values:
Calories: 232kcal | Fat: 14g | Protein: 12g | Carbs: 15g | Net carbs: 11g | Fiber: 4g | Cholesterol: 218mg | Sodium: 279mg | Potassium: 288mg

Air Fryer Cinnamon Apple Oatmeal

Servings: 4 | Preparation Time: 5 Minutes | Cooking time: 10 Minutes

Ingredients:

• 2.5 oz (80g) rolled oats
• 8 oz (240ml) water
• 8 oz (240ml) milk
• 1 medium apple, diced
• 2 tbsp sweetener/Stevia
• 1/2 tsp cinnamon
• Pinch of salt

Instructions:

1. Preheat the air fryer to 350°F (180°C).

2. In a mixing bowl, combine the rolled oats, water, milk, diced apple, sweetener/Stevia, cinnamon, and salt. Mix well.

3. Pour the oatmeal mixture into an air fryer-safe baking dish or a ramekin.

4. Place the baking dish or ramekin in the air fryer basket and cook for 12-15 minutes, or until the oatmeal is cooked and the apples are soft.

5. Serve hot and enjoy!

Note: Excess Use of sugar can increase sugar level, be mindful of how much sugar that you use

Nutritional values:

Calories: 254kcal | Fat: 4g | Protein: 8g | Carbs: 49g | Net carbs: 40g | Fiber: 9g | Cholesterol: 7mg | Sodium: 74mg | Potassium: 369mg

Air Fryer Breakfast Grilled Cheese

Serving: 4 | Preparation time: 10 minutes

Ingredients:

• 7.5 oz (224g) slices of low-carb bread
• 4 oz (112g) slices of American cheese
• 4 oz (120g) slices of ham
• 0.5 oz (15g) melted butter

Instructions:

1. Place two slices of low-carb bread on a cutting board. Top each slice with one slice of cheese and one slice of ham.

2. Close the sandwiches with the remaining slices of bread, pressing down gently.

3. Preheat the air fryer to 375°F (190°C).

4. Brush the sandwiches with melted butter on both sides.

5. Place the sandwiches in the air fryer basket, making sure they are not touching each other.

6. Air fryer the sandwiches for 6-8 minutes or until golden brown and crispy, flipping halfway through cooking.

7. Remove the sandwiches from the air fryer and let them cool for a minute before slicing and serving.

Nutritional values:

Calories: 390kcal | Fat: 21g | Protein: 20g | Carbs: 28g | Net carbs: 25g | Fiber: 3g | Cholesterol: 218mg | Sodium: 1092mg | Potassium: 257mg

Air Fryer Breakfast Bagel Sandwich

Serving: 4 | Preparation Time: 15 minutes

Ingredients:

• 2 low-carb bagels, sliced
• 2 oz (56g) slices of bacon
• 4 large eggs
• 2.88 oz (80g) slices of cheese
• Salt and pepper to taste
• Cooking spray

Instructions:

1. Preheat the air fryer to 350°F (175°C).

2. Place the bacon directly in the air fryer basket and cook until crispy. Remove the bacon from the air fryer and drain on paper towels.

3. Lightly toast the bagel slices by placing them directly in the air fryer for a couple of minutes until slightly crispy.

4. In a small bowl, whisk the eggs and season with salt and pepper.

5. Spray the air fryer basket with cooking spray.

6. Pour the beaten eggs into the air fryer basket and cook for 4-5 minutes, stirring occasionally, until the eggs are scrambled and cooked through.

7. Remove the scrambled eggs from the air fryer basket and set aside.

8. Place the bagel halves in the air fryer basket, cut side up.

9. Layer each bottom bagel half with a slice of cheese, cooked bacon, and scrambled eggs.

10. Place the top bagel halves on top of the fillings.

11. Air fry the assembled bagel sandwiches for 2-3 minutes or until the cheese is melted and the bagel is lightly toasted.

12. Remove from the air fryer and let it cool slightly before serving.

Nutritional values:

Calories: 482kcal | Fat: 27g | Protein: 25g | Carbs: 35g | Net carbs: 34g | Fiber: 1g | Cholesterol: 279mg | Sodium: 826mg | Potassium: 239mg

Chapter 2.
Salads

Air Fryer Roasted Salmon Salad

Serving: 4 | Preparation time: 10 min | Cooking time: 15-20 min

Ingredients:

• 16 oz (454g) salmon fillets
• 8 oz (227g) mixed salad greens
• 10 oz (283g) cherry tomatoes, halved
• 4 oz (113g) sliced cucumber
• 2 oz (57g) sliced red onion
• 4 oz (113g) sliced avocado
• 4 tbsp lemon juice
• 4 tbsp olive oil
• Salt and pepper to taste

Instructions:

1. Preheat the air fryer to 375°F (190°C).
2. Place the salmon fillets on a baking sheet lined with parchment paper.
3. Drizzle the salmon with 2 tablespoons of olive oil and sprinkle with salt and pepper.
4. Air fry the salmon in the preheated air fryer for 15-20 minutes, or until it is cooked through and flakes easily with a fork.
5. While the salmon is roasting, prepare the salad. In a large bowl, combine the mixed salad greens, cherry tomatoes, sliced cucumber, red onion, and avocado.
6. In a small bowl, whisk together the remaining 2 tablespoons of olive oil and lemon juice. Season with salt and pepper to taste.
7. Once the salmon is cooked, remove it from the air fryer and let it cool for a few minutes.
8. Break the salmon into chunks and add it to the salad.
9. Drizzle the lemon and olive oil dressing over the salad and toss gently to coat all the ingredients.
10. Divide the salad into four plates and serve.

Nutritional values:

Calories: 390 kcal | Fat: 25g | Protein: 30g | Carbs: 12g | Fiber: 6g | Sugar: 4g | Sodium: 90mg | Potassium: 414mg

Air Fryer Grilled Chicken Salad

Servings: 4 | Preparation time: 15 minutes

Ingredients:

• 15.87 oz (450g) chicken breasts, boneless and skinless
• 2 tbsp olive oil
• 1 tsp garlic powder
• 4 oz (120g) mixed greens
• 5 oz (150g) cherry tomatoes, halved
• 1.76 oz (50g) Red onion, sliced
• 1.76 oz (50g) Cucumber, sliced
• 2.00 oz (60ml) balsamic vinaigrette
• Salt and pepper, to taste

Instructions:

1. Preheat the air fryer to 375°F (190°C).
2. In a small bowl, whisk together the olive oil, garlic powder, salt, and pepper.
3. Brush the chicken breasts with the olive oil mixture and place them in the air fryer basket.
4. Air fry the chicken for 10-12 minutes or until cooked through, flipping halfway through.
5. Remove the chicken from the air fryer and let it cool for a few minutes. Then, slice it into strips.
6. In a large bowl, combine the mixed greens, cherry tomatoes, red onion, and cucumber. Toss to combine.
7. Add the sliced chicken to the salad and drizzle with balsamic vinaigrette. Toss again to coat.
8. Serve and enjoy!

Nutritional values:

Calories: 345kcal | Fat: 23g | Protein: 28g | Carbs: 9g | Net carbs: 7g | Fiber: 2g | Cholesterol: 79mg | Sodium: 407mg | Potassium: 813mg

Air Fryer Southwest Salad

Servings: 4 | Preparation Time: 20 Minutes

Ingredients:

- 12 oz (340g) mixed greens
- 4 oz (100g) black beans, drained and rinsed
- 3 oz (80g) corn kernels, fresh or frozen and thawed
- 1.5 oz (40g) diced red onion
- 7.05 oz (200g) avocado, diced
- 2.00 oz (60ml) salsa
- Juice of 1 lime
- Salt and pepper to taste

Instruction:

1. Preheat your air fryer to 375°F (190°C).
2. Rinse and pat dry the mixed greens.
3. In a large mixing bowl, combine the mixed greens, black beans, corn, and red onion. Toss gently to mix.
4. In a separate bowl, mash the avocado with a fork until smooth. Add salsa, salt, pepper and lime juice to the mashed avocado and stir well.
5. Drizzle the avocado mixture over the salad and toss gently to coat.
6. Transfer the salad mixture to the air fryer basket and air fry for 5-6 minutes until the salad is slightly crispy.
7. Serve immediately and enjoy your Southwest Salad!

Note: You can add grilled chicken, shrimp, or tofu for added protein.

Nutritional values:

Calories: 290 kcal | Fat: 17g | Protein: 9g | Carbohydrates: 29g | Fiber: 11g | Sugar: 4g | Sodium: 369mg | Potassium: 324mg

Air Fryer Greek Salad

Serving: 4 | Preparation time: 10 minutes

Ingredients:

- 8 oz (225g) large cucumber, diced
- 5 oz (150g) cherry tomatoes, halved
- 2 oz (60g) red onion, thinly sliced
- 3 oz (90ml) kalamata olives, pitted
- 4 oz (113g) feta cheese, crumbled
- 2 tbsp olive oil
- 2 tbsp red wine vinegar
- Salt and pepper to taste

Instructions:

1. Preheat the air fryer to 375°F (190°C).
2. Place the diced cucumber, cherry tomatoes, red onion, and kalamata olives in a large bowl.
3. Drizzle olive oil, salt, pepper and red wine vinegar over the vegetables and toss to combine.
4. Transfer the salad to the air fryer basket and cook for 5-7 minutes, or until the vegetables are slightly softened.
5. Remove from the air fryer and sprinkle crumbled feta cheese over the top.
6. Serve immediately.

Nutritional value:

Calories: 208kcal | Fat: 18g | Protein: 5g | Carbs: 8g | Fiber: 2g | Sugar: 4g | Cholesterol: 33mg | Sodium: 494mg | Potassium: 269mg

Air Fryer Caprese Salad

Serving: 4 | Preparation time: 10 minutes

Ingredients:

- 21.16-28.22 oz (600-800g) ripe tomatoes
- 8 oz (226g) fresh mozzarella cheese
- 0.35 oz (10g) fresh basil leaves
- 2 tbsp extra-virgin olive oil
- 2 tbsp balsamic vinegar
- Salt and pepper to taste
- Cooking spray

Instructions:

1. Preheat the air fryer to 375°F (190°C).
2. Slice the tomatoes and mozzarella cheese into approximately 1/4-inch-thick slices.
3. If desired, you can lightly spray the tomato and mozzarella slices with cooking spray to help with browning and prevent sticking in the air fryer.
4. Place the tomato and mozzarella slices in the air fryer basket, making sure they are arranged in a single layer.
5. Air fry the slices at 375°F (190°C) for about 3-5 minutes or until the cheese is melted and slightly golden, and the tomatoes are heated through.

6. Remove the tomato and mozzarella slices from the air fryer and transfer them to a serving plate.

7. Take the fresh basil leaves and place them on top of each tomato and mozzarella slice.

8. Drizzle extra virgin olive oil over the salad, making sure to coat each slice.

9. Follow by drizzling balsamic vinegar over the salad. The amount can vary depending on your preference.

10. Sprinkle salt and pepper to taste.

11. Serve the Caprese Salad immediately and enjoy!

Nutritional values:

Calories: 221kcal | Fat: 17g | Protein: 12g | Carbs: 7g | Fiber: 1g | Sugar: 5g | Cholesterol: 45mg | Sodium: 421mg | Potassium: 414mg

Air Fryer Waldorf Salad

Serving: 4 | Preparation time: 15 minutes

Ingredients:

• 11 oz (300g) diced apples
• 4 oz (120g) chopped celery
• 5 oz (150g) red grapes, halved
• 2 oz (60g) chopped walnuts
• 2 oz (60ml) Greek yogurt
• 1 tsp honey
• 1 tbsp apple cider vinegar

Instructions:

1. Preheat the air fryer to 375°F (190°C).

2. In a mixing bowl, combine the diced apples, chopped celery, halved grapes, and chopped walnuts.

3. In a separate bowl, whisk together the Greek yogurt, honey, and apple cider vinegar until smooth.

4. Pour the dressing over the apple mixture and stir to combine.

5. Transfer the salad to the air fryer basket and cook for 5-7 minutes, or until the apples and walnuts are slightly toasted and the grapes are slightly caramelized.

6. Remove the salad from the air fryer and serve immediately.

Note: Excess Use of honey can increase sugar level, be mindful of how much honey that you use

Nutritional values:

Calories: 197kcal | Fat: 10g | Protein: 4g | Carbs: 27g | Net carbs: 21g | Fiber: 6g | Sugar: 19g | Cholesterol: 0mg | Sodium: 25mg | Potassium: 384mg

Air Fryer Cobb Salad

Serving: 4 | Preparation Time: 20 Minutes

Ingredients:

• 4 oz (120g) mixed greens
• 8 oz (225g) cooked chicken breast, diced
• 2 hard-boiled eggs, chopped
• 1 avocado, diced
• 4 slices bacon, cooked and crumbled
• 2 oz (75g) cherry tomatoes, halved
• 1 oz (30g) crumbled blue cheese
• Salt and pepper, to taste

For the dressing:

• 4 oz (120ml) plain Greek yogurt
• 1 tbsp Dijon mustard
• 2 tbsp freshly squeezed lemon juice
• 2 cloves garlic, minced
• Salt and pepper, to taste

Instructions:

1. Preheat the air fryer to 375°F (190°C).

2. Arrange the diced chicken breast on the air fryer basket and cook for 5-7 minutes or until crispy.

3. In a large bowl, combine the mixed greens, chopped hard-boiled eggs, diced avocado, crumbled bacon, cherry tomatoes, and crumbled blue cheese.

4. Add the cooked chicken breast to the bowl and toss to combine.

5. In a small bowl, whisk together the Greek yogurt, lemon juice, Dijon mustard, minced garlic, salt, and pepper until well combined.

6. Drizzle the dressing over the salad and toss to coat.

7. Serve immediately.

Nutritional values:
Calories: 387kcal | Fat: 25g | Protein: 28g | Carbs: 13g | Fiber: 7g | Sugar: 4g | Cholesterol: 185mg | Sodium: 753mg | Potassium: 808mg

Air Fryer Asian Salad

Serving size: 4 | Preparation time: 10 minutes

Ingredients:

• 6.5 oz (180g) shredded cabbage
• 2 oz (60g) shredded carrots
• 0.5 oz (15g) chopped green onions
• 1 oz (28g) sliced almonds
• 0.7 oz (20g) crispy chow mein noodles
• 2 oz (60ml) sesame oil
• 1 tbsp less sodium soy sauce
• Salt and pepper, to taste

Instructions:

1. Preheat your air fryer to 375°F (190°C).
2. In a mixing bowl, combine the cabbage, carrots, and green onions.
3. Place the almonds and chow mein noodles in the air fryer basket and cook for 2-3 minutes or until crispy.
4. Add the crispy almonds and chow mein noodles to the mixing bowl with the vegetables.
5. In a small bowl, whisk together the sesame oil, salt, pepper and soy sauce. Pour the dressing over the salad and toss to combine.
6. Serve immediately.

Nutritional values:
Calories: 165kcal | Fat: 10g | Protein: 4g | Carbs: 16g | Net carbs: 12g | Fiber: 4g | Cholesterol: 0mg | Sodium: 415mg | Potassium: 254mg

Air Fryer Beet and Goat Cheese Salad

Serving: 4 | Preparation time: 10-15 minutes

Ingredients:

• 24 oz (680g) medium beets, trimmed and peeled
• 1 tbsp olive oil
• 2 oz (60g) mixed greens
• 1 oz (30g) crumbled goat cheese
• 1 oz (28g) chopped walnuts
• 1 tbsp balsamic vinegar
• Salt and pepper to taste

Instructions:

1. Preheat the air fryer to 400°F (200°C).
2. Cut the beets into bite-sized pieces and toss with olive oil.
3. Place the beets in a single layer in the air fryer basket and cook for 15-20 minutes, until tender.
4. In a large bowl, combine the cooked beets, mixed greens, goat cheese, and walnuts.
5. Drizzle with balsamic vinegar and toss to combine.
6. Season with salt and pepper to taste.
7. Serve immediately.

Note: You can use any type of greens you prefer in this salad, such as spinach or arugula.

Nutritional values:
Calories: 200kcal | Fat: 12g | Protein: 7g | Carbs: 19g | Net carbs: 14g | Fiber: 5g | Cholesterol: 11mg | Sodium: 227mg | Potassium: 637mg

Air Fryer Kale Salad

Serving: 4 | Preparation time: 15 minutes

Ingredients:

• 12 oz (360g) chopped kale
• 1.2 oz (40g) chopped red onion
• 1.2 oz (40g) dried cranberries
• 1 oz (28g) chopped walnuts
• 1 oz (30g) crumbled feta cheese
• 2 tbsp olive oil
• 2 tbsp balsamic vinegar
• Salt and pepper to taste

Instructions:

1. Preheat the air fryer to 375°F (190°C).
2. In a mixing bowl, combine the chopped kale, red onion, dried cranberries, and walnuts.
3. Drizzle olive oil and balsamic vinegar over the mixture, and season with salt and pepper to taste.
4. Mix everything together until the kale is coated evenly.
5. Transfer the mixture into the air fryer basket, and cook for 5-7 minutes until the kale is crispy.

6. Remove from the air fryer and sprinkle crumbled feta cheese over the top.
7. Serve and enjoy!

Nutritional values:
Calories: 189kcal | Fat: 14g | Protein: 5g | Carbs: 14g | Net carbs: 10g | Fiber: 4g | Cholesterol: 8mg | Sodium: 165mg | Potassium: 443mg

Air Fryer Taco Salad

Serving: 4 | Preparation Time: 15 minutes

Ingredients:
• 16 oz (454g) ground beef
• 1 oz (28g) 1 packet taco seasoning
• 2 oz (60ml) water
• 12 oz (360g) head romaine lettuce, chopped
• 15 oz (400g) black beans, drained and rinsed
• 2.5 oz (75g) cherry tomatoes, halved
• 1.2 oz (40g) red onion, chopped
• 1 oz (28g) low-carb tortilla strips
• Salt and Pepper to taste
• Optional toppings: avocado, salsa, sour cream

Instructions:
1. Preheat the air fryer to 400°F (200°C).
2. In a skillet over medium-high heat, cook the ground beef until browned and crumbled.
3. Stir in the taco seasoning, salt, pepper and water, and simmer for 2-3 minutes until the liquid is absorbed.
4. In a large bowl, toss together the romaine lettuce, black beans, cherry tomatoes, and red onion.
5. Add the cooked beef to the salad and toss to combine.
6. Top the salad with tortilla strips.
7. Air fry for 2-3 minutes until the tortilla strips are crispy.
8. Serve the salad with optional toppings like avocado, salsa, and sour cream.

Note: Make sure to keep an eye on the tortilla strips to prevent burning in the air fryer. You can also add other toppings like diced jalapeños or cilantro for extra flavor.

Nutritional values:
Calories: 358 | fat: 19g | Saturated fat: 6g | Cholesterol: 63mg | Sodium: 1088mg | Carbohydrates: 23g | Dietary Fiber: 7g |

Air Fryer Antipasto Salad

Serving: 4 | Preparation Time: 10 Minutes

Ingredients:
• 4 oz (120g) mixed salad greens
• 4 oz (113g) sliced salami, chopped
• 4 oz (113g) sliced pepperoni, chopped
• 4 oz (113g) fresh mozzarella cheese, cubed
• 2 oz (60g) sliced black olives
• 2 oz (60g) sliced pepperoncini peppers
• 1 oz (30g) diced red onion
• 2 oz (60ml) Italian dressing
• Salt and Pepper to Taste

Instruction:
1. Preheat the air fryer to 375°F (190°C).
2. Add the salami and pepperoni to the air fryer basket and cook for 5 minutes or until crispy.
3. In a large bowl, combine the mixed greens, crispy salami and pepperoni, fresh mozzarella cheese, black olives, pepperoncini peppers, salt, pepper and red onion.
4. Toss with Italian dressing until well coated.
5. Serve and enjoy!

Nutritional values:
Calories: 280 | Total Fat: 22g | Saturated Fat: 8g | Cholesterol: 44mg | Sodium: 1100mg | Total Carbohydrates: 8g | Dietary Fiber: 2g | Sugars: 2g | Protein: 14g

Air Fryer Mediterranean Salad

Serving: 4 | Preparation time: 10 minutes]

Ingredients:
• 7 oz (200g) head of romaine lettuce, chopped
• 2.5 oz (75g) chopped cucumber
• 2.5 oz (80g) chopped red onion
• 2.5 oz (75g) chopped cherry tomatoes
• 2.5 oz (75g) pitted kalamata olives
• 2.5 oz (75g) crumbled feta cheese
• 2 oz (60ml) extra-virgin olive oil

- 2 tbsp red wine vinegar
- Salt and black pepper, to taste

Instructions:

1. Preheat the air fryer to 400°F (200°C).
2. Add the chopped cucumber and red onion to the air fryer basket and cook for 5-7 minutes, until slightly charred and softened.
3. In a large bowl, combine the romaine lettuce, cherry tomatoes, kalamata olives, and crumbled feta cheese.
4. Add the cooked cucumber and red onion to the bowl and toss to combine.
5. In a small bowl, whisk together the extra-virgin olive oil and red wine vinegar. Season with salt and black pepper, to taste.
6. Drizzle the dressing over the salad and toss to coat.
7. Serve and enjoy!

Nutritional values:

Calories: 197 kcal | Fat: 16 g | Carbohydrates: 10 g | Fiber: 4 g | Protein: 6 g | Sugar: 4 g | Cholesterol: 20mg | Sodium: 463mg | Potassium: 540mg

Air Fryer Smoked Salmon and Avocado Salad

Serving: 4 | Preparation Time: 10 minutes

Ingredients:

- 8 oz (225g) smoked salmon, sliced
- 2 ripe avocados, sliced
- 2 oz (60g) mixed salad greens
- 1 oz (30g) red onion, thinly sliced
- 2 oz (60g) cherry tomatoes, halved
- 2 tbsp lemon juice
- 2 tbsp extra virgin olive oil
- Salt and pepper to taste
- Fresh dill, for garnish (optional)

Instructions:

1. Preheat your air fryer to 400°F (200°C) for a few minutes.
2. While the air fryer is preheating, prepare the salad ingredients. Slice the smoked salmon, avocados, and red onion. Halve the cherry tomatoes. Wash and dry the mixed salad greens.
3. In a large bowl, combine the mixed salad greens, sliced red onion, and halved cherry tomatoes.
4. Drizzle the lemon juice and extra virgin olive oil over the salad ingredients. Add salt and pepper to taste. Toss everything gently to combine.
5. Place the sliced smoked salmon in a single layer on the air fryer basket or tray.
6. Air fry the salmon at 400°F (200°C) for about 3-5 minutes until it crisps up slightly. Keep a close eye on it to prevent overcooking, as it can dry out quickly.
7. Remove the salmon from the air fryer.
8. Arrange the crispy salmon and sliced avocados on top of the salad.
9. Garnish the salad with fresh dill, if desired.
10. Serve immediately and enjoy your Air Fryer Smoked Salmon and Avocado Salad!

Nutritional values:

Calories: 250kcal | Fat: 18g | Protein: 15g | Carbohydrates: 10g | Fiber: 6g | Cholesterol: 20mg | Sodium: 620mg | Potassium: 780mg

Air Fryer Grilled Halloumi Salad

Serving: 4 | Preparation Time: 10 minutes

Ingredients:

- 8 oz (225g) Halloumi cheese, sliced
- 4 oz (120g) mixed salad greens (e.g., lettuce, spinach, arugula)
- 2 oz (60g) cherry tomatoes, halved
- 2 oz (60g) cucumber, sliced
- 2 oz (60g) red onion, thinly sliced
- 2 oz (60g) Kalamata olives, pitted and halved
- 2 tbsp extra-virgin olive oil
- 1 tbsp balsamic vinegar
- 1 tsp dried oregano
- Salt and pepper to taste
- Fresh basil leaves, for garnish (optional)

Instructions:

1. Preheat your air fryer to 390°F (200°C).
2. In a bowl, toss the salad greens, cherry tomatoes, cucumber, red onion, and Kalamata olives together to create the salad base.

3. In a separate bowl, whisk together the extra-virgin olive oil, balsamic vinegar, dried oregano, salt, and pepper to make the dressing.

4. For the Air Fryer Grilled Halloumi: Lightly brush or spray the Halloumi cheese slices with olive oil. Place the slices in the air fryer basket in a single layer.

5. Air fry the Halloumi at 390°F (200°C) for 3-4 minutes per side, or until it develops a golden-brown crust.

6. Once the Halloumi is grilled, remove from the air fryer and let it cool slightly before cutting it into bite-sized pieces.

7. Add the grilled Halloumi to the salad base.

8. Drizzle the dressing over the salad and gently toss everything together until well combined.

9. Garnish the salad with fresh basil leaves (if using).

Nutritional values:

Calories: 400 kcal | Fat: 30g | Saturated Fat: 11g | Trans Fat: 0g | Cholesterol: 25mg | Sodium: 1100mg | Carbohydrates: 12g | Fiber: 3g | Sugars: 5g | Protein: 20g

Soups

Air Fryer Minestrone Soup

Serving: 4 | Preparation time: 5-10 minutes

Ingredients:

- 5 oz (411g) 1 can of diced tomatoes
- 16 oz (480ml) vegetable broth
- 2 oz (56g) small pasta (such as ditalini or elbow)
- 2.5 oz (82g) canned kidney beans, drained and rinsed
- 2.5 oz (75g) frozen mixed vegetables
- 1 tsp of Italian seasoning
- Salt and pepper to taste

Instructions:

1. Preheat the air fryer to 375°F (190°C).
2. In a large bowl, mix together the diced tomatoes, vegetable broth, pasta, kidney beans, mixed vegetables, Italian seasoning, salt, and pepper.
3. Pour the mixture into the air fryer basket and cook for 15-20 minutes, stirring occasionally, until the pasta is cooked and the vegetables are tender.
4. Serve hot and enjoy!

Nutritional value:

Calories: 154 kcal | Fat: 0.7 g | Carbohydrates: 31.8 g | Fiber: 6.4 g | Protein: 7.4 g | Sodium: 723 mg |

Air Fryer Tomato Soup

Serving: 4 | Preparation time: 10 minutes | Cook time: 25 minutes

Ingredients:

- 32 oz (907g) ripe tomatoes, quartered
- 2 oz (60g) onion, chopped
- 3 cloves garlic, minced
- 1 tbsp olive oil
- 16 oz (473ml) chicken or vegetable broth
- 1 tsp salt
- 1/2 tsp black pepper

Instructions:

1. Preheat the air fryer to 375°F (190°C).
2. In a large bowl, toss the quartered tomatoes, chopped onion, minced garlic, and olive oil together until the vegetables are evenly coated.

3. Transfer the vegetables to the air fryer basket and cook for 15 minutes, shaking the basket every 5 minutes to ensure even cooking.
4. Once the vegetables are soft and slightly charred, transfer them to a blender or food processor and blend until smooth.
5. Pour the blended mixture into a large pot and add the broth, salt, and black pepper. Stir well to combine.
6. Bring the soup to a simmer over medium heat and cook for 10-15 minutes, stirring occasionally, until heated through and slightly thickened.
7. Serve hot, garnished with fresh basil or croutons if desired.

Nutritional value:

Calories: 120 | Fat: 4g | Carbohydrates: 19g | Fiber: 5g | Protein: 5g | Sodium: 790mg |

Air Fryer Chicken Noodle Soup

Serving: 4 | Preparation Time: 15 minutes | Cook Time: 25 minutes

Ingredients:

- 16 oz (450g) boneless, skinless chicken breast, cubed
- 47.34 oz (1400ml) chicken broth
- 1 oz (30g) carrots, sliced
- 2 stalks of celery, sliced
- 2 oz (60g) onion, diced
- 1 tsp of dried thyme
- 1 tsp of dried parsley
- Salt and pepper to taste
- 4 oz (110g) egg noodles

Instructions:

1. Preheat your air fryer to 375°F (190°C).
2. In a mixing bowl, combine the cubed chicken breast with dried thyme, dried parsley, salt, and pepper. Toss well to coat the chicken evenly.
3. Place the seasoned chicken breast in the air fryer basket and cook at 375°F (190°C) for 10-12 minutes, or until the chicken is cooked through and crispy. Remove from the air `fryer and set aside.

4. In the same air fryer basket, add the sliced carrots, celery, and diced onion. Cook at 375°F (190°C) for 5-7 minutes, or until the vegetables start to soften.

5. Meanwhile, in a separate pot, cook the egg noodles according to the package instructions until they are al dente. Drain and set aside.

6. Once the vegetables are softened, add the chicken broth to the air fryer basket along with the cooked chicken. Stir well to combine all the ingredients.

7. Continue cooking the soup in the air fryer at 375°F (190°C) for an additional 8-10 minutes, or until the flavors meld together and the soup is heated through.

8. Season the soup with salt and pepper to taste.

9. Remove the air fryer basket from the fryer and carefully transfer the cooked noodles to the soup. Stir gently to combine all the ingredients.

10. Ladle the chicken noodle soup into bowls and serve hot.

Nutritional values:
Calories: 280kcal | Fat: 5g | Protein: 32g | Carbs: 25g | Net carbs: 23g | Fiber: 2g | Cholesterol: 82mg | Sodium: 1085mg | Potassium: 860mg.

Air Fryer Lentil Soup

Preparation Time: 10 minutes | Cook Time: 30 minutes | Serving: 4

Ingredients:
• 7 oz (200g) green lentils, rinsed and drained
• 32 oz (950ml) Vegetable broth
• 2 oz (60g) onion, diced
• 1 oz (30g) carrots, sliced
• 2 stalks of celery, sliced
• 2 cloves of garlic, minced
• 1 tsp of ground cumin
• 1 tsp of paprika
• Salt and pepper to taste

Instructions:
1. Preheat your air fryer to 375°F (190°C).
2. In a large pot, bring the vegetable broth to a boil.

3. Add the rinsed and drained green lentils, diced onion, sliced carrots, sliced celery, minced garlic, ground cumin, paprika, salt, and pepper to the boiling broth.

4. Reduce the heat and simmer for 30 minutes or until the lentils are tender.

5. Once the lentils are tender, transfer the soup to the air fryer and cook for an additional 5 minutes to thicken.

6. Serve the lentil soup hot.

Note: This Lentil Soup recipe is a healthy and delicious soup that is perfect for a quick and easy meal. The air fryer is used to thicken the soup and give it a crispy texture. You can adjust the seasoning according to your taste. Enjoy!

Nutritional values:
Calories: 190kcal | Fat: 1g | Protein: 14g | Carbs: 33g | Net carbs: 21g | Fiber: 12g | Cholesterol: 0mg | Sodium: 880mg | Potassium: 820mg.

Air Fryer Split Pea Soup

Serving: 4 | Preparation Time: 10 minutes | Cook Time: 30 minutes

Ingredients:
• 7 oz (200g) dried split peas, rinsed and drained
• 32 oz (950ml) water
• 2 oz (60g) onion, diced
• 1 oz (30g) carrots, sliced
• 2 cloves of garlic, minced
• Salt and pepper to taste

Instructions:
1. Preheat your air fryer to 375°F (190°C). 2. In a large pot, bring the water to a boil.

3. Add the rinsed and drained split peas, diced onion, sliced carrots, minced garlic, salt, and pepper to the boiling water.

4. Reduce the heat and simmer for 30 minutes or until the split peas are tender.

5. Once the split peas are tender, transfer the soup to the air fryer and cook for an additional 5-10 minutes to thicken.

6. Serve the split pea soup hot.

Nutritional values:
Calories: 150kcal | Fat: 0g | Protein: 10g | Carbs: 29g | Net carbs: 19g | Fiber: 10g | Cholesterol: 0mg | Sodium: 10mg | Potassium: 710mg.

Air Fryer Butternut Squash Soup

Serving: 4 | Preparation Time: 10 minutes | Cook Time: 30 minutes

Ingredients:

• 7 oz (200g) butternut squash, peeled, seeded and diced
• 2 oz (60g) medium onion, diced
• 2 cloves of garlic, minced
• 32 oz (950ml) vegetable broth
• 1 tbsp of olive oil
• Salt and pepper to taste
• 1/2 tsp of ground cinnamon

Instructions:

1. Preheat your air fryer to 375°F (190°C).
2. In a large pot, sauté the diced onion and minced garlic in olive oil until the onion is soft and translucent.
3. Add the diced butternut squash, vegetable broth, ground cinnamon, salt, and pepper to the pot and stir to combine.
4. Bring the mixture to a boil, then reduce the heat and simmer for 20-25 minutes or until the butternut squash is tender.
5. Transfer the soup to the air fryer and cook for an additional 5-10 minutes to thicken.
6. Serve the butternut squash soup hot.

Nutritional values:
Calories: 110kcal | Fat: 3g | Protein: 3g | Carbs: 22g | Net carbs: 16g | Fiber: 6g | Cholesterol: 0mg | Sodium: 720mg | Potassium: 610mg.

Air Fryer Cauliflower Soup

Serving: 4 | Preparation Time: 10 minutes | Cook Time: 25 minutes

Ingredients:

• 30 oz (900g) cauliflower, chopped into florets
• 2 oz (60g) 1 medium onion, diced
• 2 cloves of garlic, minced
• 31 oz (950ml) vegetable broth
• 2 tbsp olive oil
• Salt and pepper to taste
• 1/4 tsp of ground nutmeg

Instructions:

1. Preheat your air fryer to 375°F (190°C).
2. In a large pot, sauté the diced onion and minced garlic in olive oil until the onion is soft and translucent.
3. Add the chopped cauliflower, vegetable broth, ground nutmeg, salt, and pepper to the pot and stir to combine.
4. Bring the mixture to a boil, then reduce the heat and simmer for 20-25 minutes or until the cauliflower is tender.
5. Transfer the soup to the air fryer and cook for an additional 5-10 minutes to thicken.
6. Serve the cauliflower soup hot.

Nutritional values:
Calories: 90kcal | Fat: 6g | Protein: 3g | Carbs: 9g | Net carbs: 6g | Fiber: 3g | Cholesterol: 0mg | Sodium: 850mg | Potassium: 440mg.

Air Fryer Broccoli Soup

Serving: 4 | Preparation Time: 10 minutes | Cook Time: 25 minutes

Ingredients:

• 30 oz (900g) broccoli, chopped into florets
• 2 oz (60g) 1 medium onion, diced
• 2 cloves of garlic, minced
• 31.5 oz (950ml) Vegetable broth
• 2 tbsp of olive oil
• Salt and pepper to taste
• 1/4 tsp of ground black pepper

Instructions:

1. Preheat your air fryer to 375°F (190°C).
2. In a large pot, sauté the diced onion and minced garlic in olive oil until the onion is soft and translucent.
3. Add the chopped broccoli, vegetable broth, ground black pepper, salt, and pepper to the pot and stir to combine.

4. Bring the mixture to a boil, then reduce the heat and simmer for 20-25 minutes or until the broccoli is tender.

5. Transfer the soup to the air fryer and cook for an additional 5-10 minutes to thicken.

6. Serve the broccoli soup hot.

Note: This Broccoli Soup recipe is a healthy and flavorful soup that is perfect for a quick and easy meal. The air fryer is used to thicken the soup and give it a crispy texture. You can add more or less vegetable broth according to your desired consistency. Enjoy!

Nutritional values:
Calories: 90kcal | Fat: 6g | Protein: 3g | Carbs: 9g | Net carbs: 6g | Fiber: 3g | Cholesterol: 0mg | Sodium: 850mg | Potassium: 440mg.

Air Fryer Cream of Mushroom Soup

Serving: 4 | Preparation Time: 10 minutes | Cook Time: 20 minutes

Ingredients:
• 8 oz (250g) sliced mushrooms
• 2 oz (60g) medium onion, diced
• 2 cloves of garlic, minced
• 31 oz (950ml) Vegetable broth
• 2 tbsp of olive oil
• 4 oz (120ml) Heavy cream
• Salt and pepper to taste
• 1/4 tsp of dried thyme

Instructions:
1. Preheat your air fryer to 375°F (190°C).
2. In a large pot, sauté the sliced mushrooms, diced onion, and minced garlic in olive oil until the onion is soft and translucent.
3. Add the vegetable broth, dried thyme, salt, and pepper to the pot and stir to combine.
4. Bring the mixture to a boil, then reduce the heat and simmer for 15-20 minutes or until the mushrooms are tender.
5. Using an immersion blender, blend the soup until smooth.
6. Stir in the heavy cream and mix well.

7. Transfer the soup to the air fryer and cook for an additional 5-10 minutes to thicken.

8. Serve the cream of mushroom soup hot.

Nutritional values:
Calories: 210kcal | Fat: 18g | Protein: 4g | Carbs: 9g | Net carbs: 7g | Fiber: 2g | Cholesterol: 51mg | Sodium: 870mg | Potassium: 320mg.

Air Fryer Clam Chowder

Serving: 4 | Preparation Time: 10 minutes | Cook Time: 20 minutes

Ingredients:
• 2 cans 13 oz (368g) chopped clams, drained
• 2 slices bacon, diced
• 2 oz (60g) medium onion, diced
• 15 oz (475ml) Chicken broth
• 8 oz (240ml) Heavy cream
• 8 oz (230g) diced potatoes
• Salt and pepper to taste
• 1 oz (30ml) Olive oil

Instructions:
1. Preheat your air fryer to 375°F (190°C).
2. In a large pot, cook the diced bacon until crisp. Remove with a slotted spoon and set aside.
3. Pour a little oil and add the diced onion to the pot and sauté until the onion is soft and translucent.
4. Add the diced potatoes, chicken broth, salt, and pepper to the pot and stir to combine.
5. Bring the mixture to a boil, then reduce the heat and simmer for 15-20 minutes or until the potatoes are tender.
6. In a small bowl, whisk together the heavy cream until slightly thickened.
7. Add the clams, bacon, and cream to the pot and stir to combine.
8. Transfer the soup to the air fryer and cook for an additional 5-10 minutes to thicken.
9. Serve the clam chowder hot.

Note: This recipe for Clam Chowder is a delicious and easy-to- make soup that is perfect for any occasion. The air fryer is used to thicken the soup and give it a crispy texture. You can adjust the seasoning according to your taste. Enjoy!

Nutritional values:
Calories: 352kcal | Fat: 27g | Protein: 10g | Carbs: 17g | Net carbs: 14g | Fiber: 3g | Cholesterol: 98mg | Sodium: 836mg | Potassium: 519mg.

Air Fryer Chicken Tortilla Soup

Serving: 4 | Preparation Time: 10 minutes | Cook Time: 20 minutes

Ingredients:

• 15 oz (450g) boneless, skinless chicken breasts, cooked and shredded
• 14 oz (400g) diced tomatoes
• 4 oz (120g) diced green chilies
• 33 oz (960ml) chicken broth
• 1 tsp ground cumin
• 1 tsp chili powder
• 1/2 tsp salt
• 1/4 tsp black pepper
• Cooking spray
• 4 low-carb tortillas cut into thin strips

Instructions:

1. Preheat your air fryer to 375°F (190°C).
2. In a large bowl, combine the cooked and shredded chicken, diced tomatoes, diced green chilies, chicken broth, ground cumin, chili powder, salt, and black pepper. Stir to thoroughly combine all the ingredients.
3. Transfer the chicken and broth mixture into the air fryer basket. Make sure not to overfill it to allow proper air circulation during cooking.
4. Cook the soup in the air fryer at 375°F (190°C) for 10-15 minutes, stirring occasionally, until the flavors meld together and the soup is heated through.
5. Meanwhile, spread the low-carb tortilla strips in a single layer on a plate or on a parchment paper-lined tray. Lightly spray the strips with cooking spray to help them turn crispy.
6. After the soup is ready, remove it from the air fryer, and set it aside.
7. Place the tortilla strips in the air fryer basket and cook at 375°F (190°C) for 5-7 minutes, or until they become crispy and golden brown. Keep an eye on them to avoid burning.
8. To serve, ladle the hot chicken tortilla soup into bowls and top each serving with the crispy tortilla strips.
9. Enjoy your delicious and flavorful Chicken Tortilla Soup, made entirely in your air fryer!

Nutritional values:
Calories: 236kcal | Fat: 4g | Protein: 34g | Carbs: 14g | Net carbs: 11g | Fiber: 3g | Cholesterol: 81mg | Sodium: 1172mg | Potassium: 789mg.

Air Fryer French Onion Soup

Serving: 4 | Preparation Time: 10 minutes | Cook Time: 25 minutes

Ingredients:

• 2 large onions, sliced
• 16 oz (475ml) Beef broth
• 2 tbsp olive oil
• 1 tbsp butter
• 1 tsp thyme
• 1/2 tsp salt
• 1/4 tsp black pepper
• 4 slices of low-carb baguette
• 2.5 oz (50g) shredded Gruyere cheese

Instructions:

1. Preheat your air fryer to 375°F (190°C).
2. In a large pot, melt the butter and olive oil over medium heat.
3. Add the onions and sauté for 10-15 minutes, until the onions are caramelized.
4. Add the beef broth, thyme, salt, and pepper to the pot and bring to a boil. Reduce heat and let it simmer for 10 minutes.
5. Meanwhile, place the slices of baguette in the air fryer basket and cook for 3-5 minutes, or until crispy and golden brown.
6. Ladle the soup into oven-safe bowls and place a slice of baguette on top of each bowl.
7. Sprinkle the shredded Gruyere cheese over the baguette slices.
8. Place the bowls in the air fryer and cook for 5-7 minutes, or until the cheese is melted and bubbly.
9. Serve hot.

Nutritional values:
Calories: 155kcal | Fat: 10g | Protein: 6g | Carbs: 12g | Net carbs: 9g | Fiber: 3g | Cholesterol: 21mg | Sodium: 661mg | Potassium: 264mg.

Air Fryer Gazpacho

Serving: 4 | Preparation Time: 10 minutes

Ingredients:

- 14 oz (400g) large tomatoes, cored and roughly chopped
- 3 oz (85g) small cucumber, peeled and roughly chopped
- 2 oz (55g) red onion, roughly chopped
- 2 oz (55g) red bell pepper, roughly chopped
- 1 garlic clove, minced
- 1 tbsp red wine vinegar
- 1 tbsp olive oil
- Salt and black pepper, to taste

Instructions:

1. Preheat your air fryer to 375°F (190°C).
2. Core the tomatoes and cut them into quarters. Place the tomato quarters in the air fryer basket.
3. Cut the cucumber, red bell pepper, and red onion into chunks. Add them to the air fryer basket with the tomatoes.
4. Place the garlic cloves (with the skin on) in the air fryer basket as well.
5. Air fry the vegetables at 375°F (190°C) for about 10-12 minutes until they are softened and slightly charred.
6. Once the vegetables are done, remove them from the air fryer and let them cool for a few minutes.
7. Peel the garlic cloves and add them to a blender or food processor along with the air-fried tomatoes, cucumber, red bell pepper, and red onion.
8. Blend the vegetables until smooth and well combined.
9. While the blender is running, drizzle in the extra virgin olive oil and red wine vinegar. Continue blending until the mixture is well emulsified.
10. Season the gazpacho with salt and pepper to taste. Adjust the seasonings according to your preference.
11. Transfer the gazpacho to a large bowl or container and refrigerate for at least 1 hour to allow the flavors to meld together and the soup to chill.
12. Once chilled, give the gazpacho a stir and taste again to adjust the seasonings if needed.
13. Serve the gazpacho in chilled bowls or glasses. You can garnish it with diced cucumber, diced tomato, or chopped fresh herbs for added flavor and presentation.

Nutritional values:
Calories: 54kcal | Fat: 3g | Protein: 1g | Carbs: 6g | Net carbs: 4g | Fiber: 2g | Sugar: 4g

Air Fryer Creamy Tomato Basil Soup

Serving: 4 | Preparation Time: 20 minutes

Ingredients:

- 28 oz (800g) canned whole peeled tomatoes
- 1 tbsp olive oil
- 2 oz (55g) onion, chopped
- 2 garlic cloves, minced
- 4 oz (120ml) Vegetable broth
- 2 oz (60g) Heavy cream
- 2 tbsp chopped fresh basil leaves
- Salt and black pepper, to taste

Instructions:

1. Preheat the air fryer to 350°F (175°C).
2. Drain the canned tomatoes, reserving the juice.
3. Add the drained tomatoes and olive oil to the air fryer basket. Air fry for 10 minutes, stirring occasionally.
4. Add the chopped onion and minced garlic to the air fryer basket. Air fry for an additional 5 minutes.
5. Add the vegetable broth and reserved tomato juice to the air fryer basket. Air fry for an additional 5 minutes.
6. Remove the air fryer basket and carefully transfer the contents to a blender or food processor.
7. Blend until smooth.
8. Return the soup to the air fryer basket and add the heavy cream, chopped basil, salt, and black pepper. Air fry for an additional 5 minutes.
9. Serve hot.

Nutritional values:

Calories: 118kcal | Fat: 7g | Protein: 3g | Carbs: 12g | Net carbs: 9g | Fiber: 3g | Sugar: 7g

Air Fryer Broccoli Cheddar Soup

Serving: 4 | Preparation Time: 10 minutes | Cooking Time: 20 minutes

Ingredients:

• 4 oz (120g) broccoli florets

• 1 oz (30g) onion, chopped

• 2 cloves garlic, minced

• 4 oz (120ml) vegetable broth

• 4 oz (120ml) milk

• 2 oz (30g) cheddar cheese

• Salt and pepper to taste

• Cooking spray

Instructions:

1. Preheat the air fryer to 375°F (190°C).

2. Lightly spray the air fryer basket with cooking spray.

3. Place the broccoli florets, chopped onion, and minced garlic in the air fryer basket. Cook for 10 minutes, shaking the basket or stirring the vegetables halfway through, until the broccoli is tender and lightly charred.

4. In a saucepan over medium heat, combine the cooked broccoli, onion, and garlic with the vegetable broth.

5. Using an immersion blender or regular blender, blend the soup until smooth, or leave some chunks of broccoli for texture if desired.

6. Return the soup to the stovetop over low heat.

7. Stir in the milk and shredded cheddar cheese until the cheese is melted and incorporated into the soup.

8. Season with salt and pepper to taste.

9. Cook the soup for an additional 5 minutes, stirring occasionally, to allow the flavors to meld together.

10. Serve the Air Fryer Broccoli Cheddar Soup hot.

Nutritional values:

Calories: 230kcal | Fat: 13g | Protein: 12g; Carbohydrates: 18g | Fiber: 4g | Cholesterol: 35mg | Sodium: 620mg | Potassium: 560mg

Chapter 3.
Vegetable side dishes

Air Fryer Roasted Broccoli

Servings: 4 | Preparation time: 5 minutes | Cooking time: 10-12 minutes

Ingredients:

- 15 oz (450g) broccoli, cut into florets
- 2 tbsp olive oil
- 1 tsp garlic powder
- 1/2 tsp salt
- 1/4 tsp black pepper
- 1 tbsp lemon juice

Instructions:

1. Preheat the air fryer to 400°F (200°C).
2. In a large bowl, toss the broccoli florets with olive oil, garlic powder, salt, and black pepper.
3. Place the seasoned broccoli in the air fryer basket in a single layer.
4. Cook for 8-10 minutes or until the broccoli is tender and slightly charred.
5. Once done, remove from the air fryer and toss with lemon juice.
6. Serve hot as a side dish.

Nutritional values:

Calories: 110kcal | Fat: 8g | Protein: 4g | Carbs: 8g | Net carbs: 5g | Fiber: 3 g | Cholesterol: 0mg | Sodium: 350mg | Potassium: 420mg

Air Fryer Garlic Herb Sweet Potato Fries

Servings: 4 | Preparation time: 10 minutes | Cooking time: 10-12 minutes

Ingredients:

- 14 oz (400g) sweet potatoes cut into fries
- 2 tbsp olive oil
- 2 tsp dried parsley
- 1 tsp garlic powder
- 1/2 tsp dried oregano
- 1/2 tsp dried thyme
- 1/4 tsp salt
- 1/4 tsp black pepper

Instructions:

1. Preheat the air fryer to 400°F (200°C).
2. In a large bowl, combine the sweet potato fries, olive oil, parsley, garlic powder, oregano, thyme, salt, and pepper. Toss until the fries are evenly coated with the seasonings.
3. Place the seasoned fries in the air fryer basket in a single layer. Cook for 10-12 minutes, flipping the fries halfway through cooking, until they are crispy and golden brown.
4. Serve immediately and enjoy!

Nutritional values:

Calories: 140kcal | Fat: 7g | Protein: 1g | Carbs: 18g | Net carbs: 15g | Fiber: 3g | Cholesterol: 0mg | Sodium: 165mg | Potassium: 320mg

Air Fryer Roasted Root Vegetables

Serving: 4 | Preparation time: 10 minutes | Cooking time: 15-20 minutes

Ingredients:

- 7 oz (200g) sweet potato, peeled and chopped into small pieces
- 3 oz (80g) medium carrot, peeled and chopped into small pieces
- 2.5 oz (70g) small parsnip, peeled and chopped into small pieces
- 3.5 oz (100g) small beet, peeled and chopped into small pieces
- 1/2 tsp dried thyme
- 1/2 tsp garlic powder
- 1 tbsp olive oil
- Salt and black pepper to taste

Instructions:

1. Preheat the air fryer to 375°F (190°C).

2. In a mixing bowl, toss the chopped vegetables with olive oil, garlic powder, dried thyme, salt, and black pepper until evenly coated.

3. Transfer the seasoned vegetables to the air fryer basket.

4. Cook for 15-20 minutes, shaking the basket every 5 minutes, or until the vegetables are tender and crispy.

5. Serve hot and enjoy!

Nutritional values:

Calories: 90 kcal | Fat: 3.8 g | Protein: 1.7 g | Carbs: 14 g | Net carbs: 11 g | Fiber: 3 g | Cholesterol: 0 mg | Sodium: 70 mg | Potassium: 355 mg

Air Fryer Brussels sprouts

Servings: 4 | Preparation time: 10 minutes | Cooking time: 12 minutes

Ingredients:

• 15 oz (450g) Brussels sprouts

• 2 tbsp olive oil

• 1/2 tsp salt

• 1/4 tsp black pepper

• 1/4 tsp garlic powder

Instructions:

1. Preheat the air fryer to 375°F (190°C).

2. Trim and halve the Brussels sprouts.

3. In a bowl, toss the Brussels sprouts with olive oil, salt, pepper, and garlic powder until evenly coated.

4. Place the Brussels sprouts in a single layer in the air fryer basket.

5. Cook for 10-12 minutes, shaking the basket every 5 minutes, until the Brussels sprouts are crispy and golden brown.

6. Serve hot.

Nutritional values:

Calories: 90kcal | Fat: 6g | Protein: 3g | Carbs: 8g | Net carbs: 5g | Fiber: 3g | Cholesterol: 0mg | Sodium: 300mg | Potassium: 370mg

Air Fryer Cauliflower Tots

Servings: 4 | Preparation time: 15 minutes

Ingredients:

• 28.2 oz (800g) head of cauliflower

• 1 egg

• 1.88 oz (50g) almond flour

• 0.88 oz (25g) grated parmesan cheese

• 1/2 tsp garlic powder

• 1/2 tsp onion powder

• Salt and pepper to taste

Instructions:

1. Preheat the air fryer to 375°F (190°C).

2. Cut the cauliflower into small florets and steam until tender.

3. In a large mixing bowl, add the steamed cauliflower and mash with a fork.

4. Add the egg, almond flour, parmesan cheese, garlic powder, onion powder, salt, and pepper. Mix until well combined.

5. Scoop about 1 tablespoon of the mixture and roll it into a tot shape.

6. Place the tots in the air fryer basket and cook for 10-12 minutes or until crispy and golden brown.

7. Serve hot with your favorite dipping sauce.

Nutritional values:

Calories: 104kcal | Fat: 6g | Protein: 7g | Carbs: 8g | Net carbs: 5g | Fiber: 3 g | Cholesterol: 47mg | Sodium: 133mg | Potassium: 371mg

Air Fryer Roasted Asparagus

Serving: 4 | Preparation time: 10 Minutes

Ingredients:

• 15 oz (450g) asparagus, trimmed

• 2 tbsp olive oil

• 1/2 tsp garlic powder

• Salt and pepper to taste

Instructions:

1. Preheat the air fryer to 400°F (200°C) for 5 minutes.

2. In a bowl, toss the asparagus with olive oil, garlic powder, salt, and pepper.

3. Place the asparagus in the air fryer basket in a single layer.

4. Air fry for 6-8 minutes or until the asparagus is tender and slightly crispy.

5. Serve hot.

Nutritional values:
Calories: 90kcal | Fat: 6g | Protein: 3g | Carbs: 8g | Net carbs: 4g | Fiber: 4g | Cholesterol: 0mg | Sodium: 150mg | Potassium: 484mg

Air Fryer Quinoa Cakes

Serving: 4 | Preparation Time: 15 minutes | Cooking Time: 20 minutes

Ingredients:

• 6 oz (180g) cooked quinoa
• 2 oz (60g) grated zucchini
• 1 oz (30g) grated carrot
• 1 oz (30g) chopped spinach or kale
• 1 oz (30g) diced red bell pepper
• 1 oz (30g) diced onion
• 1 oz (30g) shredded cheddar cheese
• 2 large eggs
• 2 tbsp low-carb breadcrumbs
• 1 tsp dried herbs (such as oregano or thyme)
• Salt and pepper to taste
• Cooking spray

Instructions:

1. Preheat the air fryer to 375°F (190°C).
2. In a large bowl, combine the cooked quinoa, grated zucchini, grated carrot, chopped spinach or kale, diced red bell pepper, diced onion, shredded cheddar cheese, eggs, breadcrumbs, dried herbs, salt, and pepper. Mix well until all ingredients are evenly incorporated.
3. Using your hands, shape the mixture into round patties, about 2-3 inches in diameter.
4. Lightly spray the air fryer basket with cooking spray to prevent sticking.
5. Place the quinoa cakes in a single layer in the air fryer basket.
6. Cook in the air fryer at 375°F (190°C) for 10 minutes, flipping the cakes halfway through, until they are golden brown and crispy.
7. Once cooked, remove the quinoa cakes from the air fryer and let them cool slightly before serving.
8. Serve the Air Fryer Quinoa Cakes as a nutritious and flavorful appetizer or side dish.

Nutritional values:
Calories: 170kcal | Fat: 7g | Protein: 9g | Carbohydrates: 19g | Fiber: 3g | Cholesterol: 105mg | Sodium: 250mg | Potassium: 270mg

Air Fryer Carrot Chips

Serving size: 4 servings | Preparation time: 10 minutes | Cooking time: 8-10 minutes

Ingredients:

• 8 oz (240g) carrots, peeled and sliced into thin chips
• 1 tbsp olive oil
• 1/2 tbsp garlic powder
• 1/2 tsp paprika
• Salt and pepper, to taste

Instructions:

1. Preheat the air fryer to 375°F (190°C).
2. In a large mixing bowl, combine the sliced carrots, olive oil, garlic powder, paprika, salt, and black pepper. Toss well to evenly coat the carrots.
3. Place the coated carrot slices in the air fryer basket in a single layer. Do not overcrowd.
4. Air fry for 8-10 minutes or until the carrot chips are golden brown and crispy.
5. Remove from the air fryer and serve hot.

Nutritional values:
Calories: 70kcal | Fat: 3.5g | Protein: 1g | Carbs: 9g | Net carbs: 6g | Fiber: 3g | Cholesterol: 0mg | Sodium: 200mg | Potassium: 330mg

Air Fryer Butternut Squash Fries

Servings: 2-4 | Preparation time: 10-15 minutes

Ingredients:

• 24 oz (600g) butternut squash, peeled and sliced into fry shapes
• 1 tbsp olive oil
• 1 tsp paprika
• 1 tsp garlic powder
• Salt and pepper to taste

Instructions:

1. Preheat the air fryer to 375°F (190°C).

2. Toss the butternut squash fries with olive oil, paprika, garlic powder, salt, and pepper in a bowl.
3. Place the seasoned butternut squash fries into the air fryer basket in a single layer.
4. Cook for 10-12 minutes or until crispy, flipping the fries halfway through cooking.
5. Remove from the air fryer and serve immediately.

Nutritional values:

Calories: 98kcal | Fat: 3.5g | Protein: 2g | Carbs: 19g | Net carbs: 16g | Fiber: 3g | Cholesterol: 0mg | Sodium: 167mg | Potassium: 649mg

Air Fryer Green Beans

Servings: 4 | Preparation time: 10 minutes

Ingredients:

- 15 oz (450 g) fresh green beans, washed and trimmed
- 1 tbsp olive oil
- 1 tsp garlic powder, paprika, dried herbs
- 1/2 tsp salt
- 1/4 tsp black pepper

Instructions:

1. Preheat the air fryer to 400°F (200°C).
2. In a large mixing bowl, toss the green beans with olive oil, paprika, dried herbs, garlic powder, salt, and black pepper until evenly coated.
3. Transfer the seasoned green beans to the air fryer basket.
4. Air fry for 8-10 minutes, shaking the basket halfway through, until the green beans are crispy and tender.
5. Serve hot and enjoy!

Nutritional values:

Calories: 75kcal | Fat: 4g | Protein: 2g | Carbs: 9g | Net carbs: 6g | Fiber: 3g | Cholesterol: 0mg | Sodium: 305mg | Potassium: 300mg

Dairy Products Recipe

Air Fryer Mozzarella Sticks

Servings: 4 | Preparation time: 15 minutes

Ingredients:

• 8 oz (225g) mozzarella cheese cut into sticks
• 1 oz (30g) almond flour
• 0.7 oz (22g) grated parmesan cheese
• 1 tsp garlic powder
• 1 tsp onion powder
• 1 tsp dried oregano
• 1/2 tsp salt
• 2 large eggs, beaten
• Marinara Sauce

Instructions:

1. Preheat the air fryer to 400°F (200°C).
2. In a small bowl, mix together the almond flour, parmesan cheese, garlic powder, onion powder, oregano, and salt.
3. Dip each mozzarella stick into the beaten eggs, then coat with the almond flour mixture.
4. Place the coated mozzarella sticks in the air fryer basket, making sure they are not touching each other.
5. Air fry for 5-6 minutes or until golden brown and crispy.
6. Serve hot with marinara sauce.

Nutritional values:
Calories: 225kcal | Fat: 17g | Protein: 17g | Carbs: 5g | Net carbs: 3g | Fiber: 2g | Cholesterol: 122mg | Sodium: 667mg | Potassium: 63mg

Air Fryer Grilled Cheese Sandwich

Serving: 4 | Preparation time: 10 minutes | Cooking time: 5-7 minutes

Ingredients:

• 9.6 oz (272g) low-carb bread (such as Ezekiel bread)
• 1.88 oz (56g) shredded cheddar cheese
• 1.88 oz (56g) shredded mozzarella cheese
• 2 tbsp unsalted butter, softened
• 1/4 tsp garlic powder
• 1/4 tsp onion powder

Instructions:

1. Preheat the air fryer to 375°F (190°C).
2. In a bowl, mix the cheddar cheese, mozzarella cheese, butter, garlic powder, and onion powder.
3. Spread the mixture evenly on 4 slices of bread, then top each with the remaining bread slices.
4. Place the sandwiches in the air fryer basket and cook for 5-7 minutes or until the cheese is melted and the bread is toasted.
5. Serve hot.

Nutritional values:
Calories: 320kcal | Fat: 21g | Protein: 19g | Carbs: 16g | Net carbs: 10g | Fiber: 6g | Cholesterol: 60mg | Sodium: 540mg | Potassium: 144mg

Air Fryer Cheesy Garlic Bread

Servings: 4 | Preparation time: 5 minutes | Cooking time: 5-7 minutes

Ingredients:

• 6.4 oz (180g) slices of low-carb bread (such as Ezekiel bread)
• 2 tbsp unsalted butter, softened
• 1/4 tsp dried oregano
• 1/4 tsp dried basil
• 1/4 tsp dried parsley
• 1/4 shredded mozzarella cheese
• 2 tbsp grated parmesan cheese
• 1 garlic clove, minced

Instructions:

1. Preheat the air fryer to 375°F (190°C).
2. In a small bowl, mix the butter, minced garlic, oregano, basil, and parsley.
3. Spread the butter mixture evenly on each slice of bread.
4. Top each slice with mozzarella and parmesan cheese.

5. Place the bread slices in the air fryer basket and cook for 5-7 minutes or until the cheese is melted and the bread is toasted.
6. Serve hot.

Nutritional values:

Calories: 180kcal | Fat: 13g | Protein: 8g | Carbs: 9g | Net carbs: 5g | Fiber: 4g | Cholesterol: 35mg | Sodium: 300mg | Potassium: 72mg

Air Fryer Cream Cheese Stuffed Jalapenos

Serving: 4 | Preparation time: 15 minutes | Cooking time: 12 minutes

Ingredients:

- 8 oz (249g) Jalapenos, halved lengthwise and seeded
- 1/4 tsp garlic powder
- 4 oz (115g) cream cheese, softened
- 1/4 tsp onion powder
- 1.8 oz (50g) shredded cheddar cheese
- Salt and pepper to taste
- 1.8 oz (50g) almond flour
- 1 large egg, beaten

Instructions:

1. Preheat the air fryer to 375°F (190°C).
2. In a bowl, mix the cream cheese, cheddar cheese, garlic powder, onion powder, salt, and pepper until well combined.
3. Fill each jalapeno half with the cream cheese mixture.
4. In a shallow dish, combine the almond flour and beaten egg.
5. Dip each stuffed jalapeno half into the egg mixture, then coat in almond flour mixture.
6. Place the stuffed jalapeno halves into the air fryer basket and cook for 12 minutes or until golden brown and crispy.
7. Serve immediately and enjoy!

Nutritional values:

Calories: 150kcal | Fat: 12g | Protein: 6g | Carbs: 6g | Net carbs: 3g | Fiber: 3g | Cholesterol: 61mg | Sodium: 160mg | Potassium: 193mg

Air Fryer Goat Cheese and Tomato Tart

Servings: 4 | Preparation time: 10 minutes | Cooking time: 15 minutes

Ingredients:

- 7 oz (200g) filo pastry, thawed
- 4 oz (115g) goat cheese, crumbled
- 7 oz (200g) large tomato, thinly sliced
- 0.4 oz (10g) fresh basil leaves, chopped
- 1/4 tsp garlic powder
- Salt and pepper to taste
- 1 tbsp. olive oil

Instructions:

1. Preheat the air fryer to 375°F (190°C).
2. Unroll the filo pastry sheet and place it onto a parchment paper-lined air fryer basket.
3. Prick the pastry all over with a fork.
4. In a bowl, mix the goat cheese, basil, garlic powder, salt, and pepper.
5. Spread the goat cheese mixture onto the filo pastry, leaving a small border around the edges.
6. Arrange the tomato slices on top of the goat cheese mixture.
7. Brush the edges of the filo pastry with olive oil.
8. Air fry the tart for 15 minutes or until the filo pastry is golden brown and the tomatoes are slightly roasted.
9. Slice the tart into squares and serve immediately.

Nutritional values:

Calories: 230kcal | Fat: 16g | Protein: 6g | Carbs: 16g | Net carbs: 12g | Fiber: 4g | Cholesterol: 15mg | Sodium: 200mg | Potassium: 220mg

Air Fryer Baked Brie with Honey and Almonds

Serving: 4 | Preparation time: 5 minutes | Cooking time: 8 minutes

Ingredients:

- 8 oz (240g) wheel of brie cheese
- 1 oz (30g) sliced almonds
- 2 tsp honey

Instructions:

1. Preheat the air fryer to 375°F (190°C).
2. Place the brie wheel in a small oven-safe dish that fits inside the air fryer basket.
3. Sprinkle the sliced almonds over the brie.
4. Drizzle the honey over the almonds and brie.
5. Place the dish with the brie into the air fryer basket.
6. Air fry for 8 minutes, or until the brie is melted and bubbly.
7. Remove the dish from the air fryer basket.
8. Serve immediately with crackers or bread.

Note: Excess Use of honey can increase sugar level, be mindful of how much honey that you use

Nutritional values:

Calories: 400kcal | Fat: 32g | Protein: 23g | Carbs: 10g | Net carbs: 10g | Fiber: 0g | Cholesterol: 100mg | Sodium: 720mg | Potassium: 180mg

Air Fryer Cheesy Broccoli

Serving: 4 | Preparation Time: 15 minutes

Ingredients:

- 10 oz (284g) broccoli florets
- 2 tbsp olive oil
- 1/2 tsp garlic powder
- 1/2 tsp onion powder
- 1/2 tsp paprika
- Salt and pepper to taste
- 2 oz (60g) shredded cheddar cheese

Instructions:

1. Preheat the air fryer to 375°F (190°C).
2. In a large bowl, toss the broccoli florets with olive oil, garlic powder, onion powder, paprika, salt, and pepper until well coated.
3. Place the seasoned broccoli florets in the air fryer basket in a single layer.
4. Air fry for 10-12 minutes, shaking the basket or flipping the broccoli halfway through, until the broccoli is tender and lightly browned.
5. Sprinkle the shredded cheddar cheese evenly over the cooked broccoli.
6. Air fry for another 2-3 minutes, or until the cheese is melted and bubbly.

7. Remove from the air fryer and serve immediately.

Nutritional values:

Calories: 160kcal | Fat: 13g | Protein: 7g | Carbs: 6g | Net carbs: 4g | Fiber: 2g | Cholesterol: 15mg | Sodium: 160mg | Potassium: 370mg

Air Fryer Parmesan Brussels sprouts

Serving: 4 | Preparation Time: 20 minutes

Ingredients:

- 15 oz (450 g) Brussels sprouts, trimmed and halved
- 2 tbsp olive oil
- 1 oz (30g) grated Parmesan cheese
- 1 tsp garlic powder
- Salt and pepper to taste

Instructions:

1. Preheat the air fryer to 400°F (200°C).
2. In a large bowl, toss the Brussels sprouts with olive oil, grated Parmesan cheese, garlic powder, salt, and pepper until well coated.
3. Place the seasoned Brussels sprouts in the air fryer basket in a single layer.
4. Air fry for 12-15 minutes, shaking the basket or tossing the Brussels sprouts halfway through, until they are crispy and golden brown.
5. Remove from the air fryer and serve immediately.

Nutritional values:

Calories: 140kcal | Fat: 9g | Protein: 6g | Carbs: 11g | Net carbs: 6g | Fiber: 5g | Cholesterol: 5mg | Sodium: 180mg | Potassium: 600mg

Air Fryer Creamy Garlic Mushrooms

Serving: 4 | Preparation Time: 20 minutes

Ingredients:

- 15 oz (450g) button mushrooms, cleaned and halved
- 2 tbsp olive oil
- 4 cloves garlic, minced
- 4 oz (120ml) heavy cream

- 2 oz (60ml) chicken or vegetable broth
- 1 oz (30g) grated Parmesan cheese
- 1 tbsp fresh thyme leaves (or 1 tsp dried thyme)
- Salt and pepper to taste
- Fresh parsley, chopped (for garnish)

Instructions:

1. Preheat your air fryer to 375°F (190°C) for a few minutes.
2. In a mixing bowl, toss the halved button mushrooms with olive oil, minced garlic, fresh thyme leaves (or dried thyme), salt, and pepper until the mushrooms are evenly coated.
3. Place the seasoned mushrooms in the air fryer basket or on the tray in a single layer.
4. Air fry the mushrooms at 375°F (190°C) for about 8-10 minutes, shaking the basket or flipping the mushrooms halfway through to ensure even cooking. The mushrooms should be tender and slightly golden.
5. Once the mushrooms are cooked, push them to one side of the air fryer basket, creating a space for the sauce.
6. In the other half of the air fryer basket, pour the heavy cream and chicken or vegetable broth.
7. Air fry the cream and broth mixture at 375°F (190°C) for about 4-5 minutes, or until it begins to simmer.
8. Add the grated Parmesan cheese to the cream and broth mixture, stirring until the cheese is melted and the sauce is smooth.
9. Carefully mix the creamy sauce with the cooked mushrooms, ensuring they are evenly coated.
10. Adjust the seasoning with additional salt and pepper if needed.
11. Garnish the creamy garlic mushrooms with chopped fresh parsley.
12. Serve the Air Fryer Creamy Garlic Mushrooms as a delicious side dish.

Nutritional values:

Calories: 220 kcal | Fat: 18g | Saturated Fat: 8g | Trans Fat: 0g | Cholesterol: 40mg | Sodium: 150mg | Carbohydrates: 8g | Fiber: 2g | Sugars: 2g | Protein: 7g

Air Fryer Ricotta Stuffed Portobello Mushrooms

Serving: 4 | Preparation Time: 20 minutes

Ingredients:

- 21 oz (600g) large Portobello mushrooms
- 8.8 oz (250g) ricotta cheese
- 1 oz (30g) grated Parmesan cheese
- 2 cloves garlic, minced
- 1 oz (30g) chopped fresh basil
- 1 oz (30g) chopped fresh parsley
- 1/2 tsp dried oregano
- Salt and pepper to taste
- Olive oil, for drizzling

Instructions:

1. Preheat the air fryer to 375°F (190°C).
2. Remove the stems from the Portobello mushrooms and gently scrape out the gills using a spoon.
3. In a bowl, combine ricotta cheese, grated Parmesan cheese, minced garlic, chopped fresh basil, chopped fresh parsley, dried oregano, salt, and pepper. Mix well.
4. Spoon the ricotta mixture into the mushroom caps, filling them evenly.
5. Drizzle the stuffed mushrooms with olive oil.
6. Place the mushrooms in the air fryer basket.
7. Air fry for 12-15 minutes, or until the mushrooms are tender and the cheese is melted and golden brown on top.
8. Remove from the air fryer and serve hot.

Nutritional values:

Calories: 210kcal | Fat: 15g | Protein: 12g | Carbs: 8g | Net carbs: 6g | Fiber: 2g | Cholesterol: 40mg | Sodium: 250mg | Potassium: 630mg

Chapter 4.
Turkey Recipes

Air Fryer Turkey Burgers

Serving: 4 | Preparation time: 5 minutes | Cooking time: 12 minutes

Ingredients:

• 15 oz (450g) pound ground turkey
• 0.8 oz (25g) almond flour
• 2 oz (60 ml) unsweetened almond milk
• 0.5 oz (15g) chopped fresh parsley
• 0.5 oz (15g) chopped red onion
• 1 tsp garlic powder
• Salt and pepper to taste

Instructions:

1. Preheat the air fryer to 375°F (190°C).
2. In a bowl, mix together the ground turkey, almond flour, almond milk, parsley, red onion, garlic powder, salt, and pepper until well combined.
3. Divide the mixture into 4 equal portions and form each portion into a patty.
4. Place the turkey patties in the air fryer basket, leaving space between them.
5. Air fry for 12 minutes, flipping the patties halfway through, until the internal temperature reaches 165°F (74°C).
6. Remove the patties from the air fryer basket and let them rest for 5 minutes before serving.
7. Serve on buns with your favorite toppings.

Nutritional values:

Calories: 200kcal | Fat: 10g | Protein: 23g | Carbs: 4g | Net carbs: 3g | Fiber: 1g | Cholesterol: 85mg | Sodium: 130mg | Potassium: 300mg

Air Fryer Turkey Meatballs

Servings: 4 | Preparation time: 10 minutes | Cooking time: 12 minutes

Ingredients:

• 15 oz (450g) ground turkey
• 0.88 oz (25g) almond flour
• 0.5 oz (15g) grated parmesan cheese
• 0.5 oz (15g) chopped fresh parsley
• 1 tsp garlic powder
• Salt and pepper to taste

Instructions:

1. Preheat the air fryer to 375°F (190°C).
2. In a bowl, mix together the ground turkey, almond flour, parmesan cheese, parsley, garlic powder, salt, and pepper until well combined.
3. Form the mixture into 16 equal-sized meatballs.
4. Place the meatballs in the air fryer basket, leaving space between them.
5. Air fry for 12 minutes, flipping the meatballs halfway through, until the internal temperature reaches 165°F (74°C).
6. Remove the meatballs from the air fryer basket and let them rest for 5 minutes before serving.
7. Serve with your favorite dipping sauce.

Nutritional values:

Calories: 130kcal | Fat: 7g | Protein: 15g | Carbs: 2g | Net carbs: 1g | Fiber: 1g | Cholesterol: 50mg | Sodium: 110mg | Potassium: 190mg

Air Fryer Turkey Breast with Garlic-Herb Butter

Serving: 4 | Preparation time: 10 minutes | Cooking time: 50 minutes

Ingredients:

• 30 oz (900g) boneless turkey breast
• 2 cloves garlic, minced
• 4 tbsp unsalted butter, at room temperature
• 1 tsp dried thyme
• 1 tsp dried rosemary
• Salt and pepper to taste

Instructions:

1. Preheat the air fryer to 350°F (175°C).
2. In a small bowl, mix together the butter, garlic, thyme, and rosemary until well combined.

3. Season the turkey breast with salt and pepper, and then spread the garlic-herb butter all over the turkey.

4. Place the turkey breast in the air fryer basket, skin-side up.

5. Air fry for 40-50 minutes, until the internal temperature of the turkey reaches 165°F (74°C).

6. Remove the turkey breast from the air fryer basket and let it rest for 10 minutes before slicing and serving.

Nutritional values:

Calories: 270kcal | Fat: 14g | Protein: 33g | Carbs: 0g | Net carbs: 0g | Fiber: 0g | Cholesterol: 120mg | Sodium: 160mg | Potassium: 390mg

Air Fryer Turkey Legs with Rosemary and Thyme

Serving: 4 | Preparation time: 10 minutes | Cooking time: 20 minutes

Ingredients:

• 30 oz (900g) turkey legs
• 2 tbsp olive oil
• 1 tbsp chopped fresh rosemary
• 1 tbsp chopped fresh thyme
• 2 cloves garlic, minced
• Salt and pepper to taste

Instructions:

1. Preheat the air fryer to 375°F (190°C).

2. In a small bowl, mix together the olive oil, rosemary, thyme, garlic, salt, and pepper.

3. Rub the mixture all over the turkey legs, making sure to coat them evenly.

4. Place the turkey legs in the air fryer basket, leaving space between them.

5. Air fry for 20 minutes, flipping the legs halfway through, until the internal temperature reaches 165°F (74°C).

6. Remove the turkey legs from the air fryer basket and let them rest for 5 minutes before serving.

Nutritional values:

Calories: 350kcal | Fat: 22g | Protein: 35g | Carbs: 1g | Net carbs: 1g | Fiber: 0g | Cholesterol: 155mg | Sodium: 260mg | Potassium: 550mg

Air Fryer Turkey Tenderloin with Mustard-Herb Crust

Serving: 4 | Preparation time: 10 minutes | Cooking time: 25-30 minutes

Ingredients:

• 15 oz (453g) turkey tenderloin
• 2 tbsp Dijon mustard
• 1 tbsp olive oil
• 1 tsp dried thyme
• 1 tsp dried rosemary
• 1 tsp garlic powder
• Salt and pepper to taste

Instructions:

1. Preheat the air fryer to 380°F (193°C).

2. In a small bowl, mix together the Dijon mustard, olive oil, dried thyme, dried rosemary, garlic powder, salt, and pepper.

3. Rub the mixture all over the turkey tenderloin; making sure it's coated evenly.

4. Place the turkey tenderloin in the air fryer basket.

5. Cook for 25-30 minutes or until the internal temperature reaches 165°F (74°C).

6. Let the turkey rest for 5 minutes before slicing and serving.

Nutritional values:

Calories: 187 kcal | Fat: 4g | Protein: 33g | Carbs: 1g | Net carbs: 1g | Fiber: 0g | Cholesterol: 82mg | Sodium: 293mg | Potassium: 407mg

Air Fryer Turkey Sausage Patties

Serving: 4 | Preparation time: 10 minutes | Cooking time: 10-12 minutes

Ingredients:

• 15 oz (453g) ground turkey
• 1 tsp salt
• 1 tsp dried sage
• 1/2 tsp black pepper
• 1/4 tsp red pepper flakes
• 1/4 tsp garlic powder

Instructions:

1. Preheat the air fryer to 375°F (190°C).
2. In a mixing bowl, combine the ground turkey, salt, dried sage, black pepper, red pepper flakes, and garlic powder.
3. Mix the ingredients thoroughly using your hands.
4. Shape the mixture into 12 patties of even size.
5. Place the patties in the air fryer basket, leaving some space between them.
6. Cook for 10-12 minutes or until the internal temperature reaches 165°F (74°C).
7. Flip the patties halfway through the cooking time.
8. Remove from the air fryer and let them rest for a minute before serving.

Nutritional values:

Calories: 87 kcal | Fat: 3g | Protein: 14g | Carbs: 0g | Net carbs: 0g | Fiber: 0g | Cholesterol: 42mg | Sodium: 328mg | Potassium: 164mg

Air Fryer Turkey Bacon Wrapped Asparagus

Serving: 4 | Preparation time: 10 minutes | Cooking time: 8-10 minutes

Ingredients:

- 16.9 oz (480g) asparagus spears
- 6.4 oz (180g) turkey bacon slices
- 1 tbsp olive oil
- Salt and black pepper, to taste
- 1 tsp dried rosemary
- 1 tsp garlic powder

Instructions:

1. Preheat the air fryer to 400°F (200°C).
2. Snap the woody ends off the asparagus and discard them.
3. Divide the asparagus spears into 6 equal portions.
4. Wrap each portion with one turkey bacon slice.
5. Brush the bacon-wrapped asparagus with olive oil.
6. Season with salt, rosemary, garlic powder and black pepper.
7. Place the asparagus bundles in the air fryer basket.

8. Cook for 8-10 minutes or until the bacon is crispy and the asparagus is tender.
9. Flip the bundles halfway through the cooking time.
10. Remove from the air fryer and let them cool for a minute before serving.

Nutritional values:

Calories: 95 kcal | Fat: 6g | Protein: 8g | Carbs: 3g | Net carbs: 2g | Fiber: 1g | Cholesterol: 23mg | Sodium: 318mg | Potassium: 246mg

Air Fryer Turkey Cutlets with Lemon and Garlic

Serving: 4 | Preparation time: 5 minutes | Cooking time: 8-10 minutes

Ingredients:

- 15 oz (453g) turkey cutlets
- 2 tbsp olive oil
- 1 tbsp lemon juice
- 1 tsp garlic powder
- 1/2 tsp dried thyme
- Salt and black pepper, to taste

Instructions:

1. Preheat the air fryer to 400°F (200°C).
2. In a small bowl, mix together the olive oil, lemon juice, garlic powder, dried thyme, salt, and black pepper.
3. Brush the turkey cutlets with the mixture on both sides.
4. Place the cutlets in the air fryer basket.
5. Cook for 8-10 minutes or until the internal temperature reaches 165°F (74°C).
6. Flip the cutlets halfway through the cooking time.
7. Remove from the air fryer and let them rest for a minute before serving.

Nutritional values:

Calories: 222 kcal | Fat: 11g | Protein: 30g | Carbs: 1g | Net carbs: 1g | Fiber: 0g | Cholesterol: 85mg | Sodium: 94mg | Potassium: 397mg

Air Fryer Turkey Drumsticks with BBQ Rub

Serving: 4 | Preparation time: 10 minutes | Cooking time: 25-30 minutes

Ingredients:

• 15 oz (450g) turkey drumsticks
• 1 tbsp olive oil
• 1 tbsp smoked paprika
• 1 tsp honey
• 1 tbsp chili powder
• 1 tsp garlic powder
• 1/2 tsp onion powder
• 1/2 tsp dried oregano
• 1/2 tsp salt
• 1/4 tsp black pepper

Instructions:

1. Preheat the air fryer to 375°F (190°C).
2. In a small bowl, mix together the smoked paprika, honey, chili powder, garlic powder, onion powder, dried oregano, salt, and black pepper.
3. Pat the turkey drumsticks dry with paper towels.
4. Rub the drumsticks with olive oil on all sides.
5. Sprinkle the BBQ rub over the drumsticks and rub it in with your hands.
6. Place the drumsticks in the air fryer basket.
7. Cook for 25-30 minutes or until the internal temperature reaches 165°F (74°C).
8. Flip the drumsticks halfway through the cooking time.
9. Remove from the air fryer and let them rest for a few minutes before serving.

Note: The use of too much sugar or honey might affect your sugar level.

Nutritional values:
Calories: 258 kcal | Fat: 12g | Protein: 34g | Carbs: 3g | Net carbs: 3g | Fiber: 0g | Cholesterol: 122mg | Sodium: 420mg | Potassium: 468mg

Air Fryer Turkey Thighs with Lemon and Thyme

Serving: 4 | Preparation time: 10 minutes | Cooking time: 25-30 minutes

Ingredients:

• 15 oz (450g) turkey thighs bone-in and skin-on
• 1 tbsp olive oil
• 1 tbsp fresh lemon juice
• 2 cloves garlic, minced
• 1 tbsp fresh thyme leaves
• 1 tsp salt
• 1/2 tsp black pepper

Instructions:

1. Preheat the air fryer to 375°F (190°C).
2. In a small bowl, mix together the olive oil, lemon juice, minced garlic, fresh thyme leaves, salt, and black pepper.
3. Pat the turkey thighs dry with paper towels.
4. Brush the turkey thighs on all sides with the lemon and thyme mixture.
5. Place the turkey thighs in the air fryer basket, skin side up.
6. Cook for 25-30 minutes or until the internal temperature reaches 165°F (74°C).
7. Flip the turkey thighs halfway through the cooking time.
8. Remove from the air fryer and let them rest for a few minutes before serving.

Nutritional values:
Calories: 287 kcal | Fat: 16g | Protein: 31g | Carbs: 2g | Net carbs: 2g | Fiber: 0g | Cholesterol: 145mg | Sodium: 652mg | Potassium: 424mg

Air Fryer Turkey Fajitas

Serving: 4 | Preparation Time: 20 minutes

Ingredients:

• 15 oz (450g) turkey breast, sliced
• 2 oz (60g) onion, sliced
• 4 oz (120g) green bell pepper, sliced
• 4 oz (120g) red bell pepper, sliced
• 1 tbsp olive oil
• 1 tbsp taco seasoning
• Juice of 1 lime
• Salt and pepper to taste

Instructions:

1. Preheat the air fryer to 380°F (193°C).

2. In a bowl, combine turkey breast, onion, green bell pepper, red bell pepper, olive oil, taco seasoning, lime juice, salt, and pepper. Mix well.

3. Place the mixture in the air fryer basket and cook for 15-20 minutes, shaking the basket occasionally.

4. Serve hot with tortillas, avocado, and any other desired toppings.

Nutritional values:

Calories: 225kcal | Fat: 7g | Protein: 35g | Carbs: 8g | Net carbs: 5g | Fiber: 3 g | Cholesterol: 82mg | Sodium: 650mg | Potassium: 715mg

Air Fryer Turkey Schnitzel

Serving: 4 | Preparation Time: 20 minutes

Ingredients:

• 15 oz (450g) turkey cutlets
• 2 oz (60g) almond flour
• 1 oz (30g) grated parmesan cheese
• 1 tsp paprika
• 1/2 tsp garlic powder
• 1/4 tsp onion powder
• 1/4 tsp dried thyme
• Salt and pepper to taste
• 1 egg, beaten
• Cooking spray

Instructions:

1. Preheat the air fryer to 400°F (204°C).

2. In a bowl, combine almond flour, parmesan cheese, paprika, garlic powder, onion powder, thyme, salt, and pepper.

3. Dip each turkey cutlet in the beaten egg, then coat in the almond flour mixture.

4. Spray the air fryer basket with cooking spray and place the turkey cutlets in a single layer.

5. Cook for 8-10 minutes, flipping halfway through, until golden brown and crispy.

6. Serve hot with your favorite dipping sauce.

Nutritional values:

Calories: 301kcal | Fat: 13g | Protein: 38g | Carbs: 4g | Net carbs: 2g | Fiber: 2 g | Cholesterol: 154mg | Sodium: 230mg | Potassium: 515mg

Air Fryer Turkey Kofta Kebabs

Serving: 4 | Preparation Time: 25 minutes

Ingredients:

• 15 oz (450g) ground turkey
• 1 oz (28g) almond flour
• 1 oz (30g) onion, finely chopped
• 2 cloves garlic, minced
• 1 tbsp olive oil
• 1 tsp ground cumin
• 1 tsp paprika
• 1/2 tsp ground coriander
• Salt and pepper to taste
• Cooking spray

Instructions:

1. Preheat the air fryer to 400°F (204°C).

2. In a bowl, combine ground turkey, almond flour, onion, garlic, olive oil, cumin, paprika, coriander, salt, and pepper.

3. Mix well and form the mixture into 8 kebab shapes.

4. Spray the air fryer basket with cooking spray and place the kebabs in a single layer.

5. Cook for 10-12 minutes, flipping halfway through, until fully cooked and golden brown.

6. Serve hot with your favorite dipping sauce and salad.

Nutritional values:

Calories: 202kcal | Fat: 12g | Protein: 21g | Carbs: 4g | Net carbs: 2g | Fiber: 2 g | Cholesterol: 83mg | Sodium: 65mg | Potassium: 340mg

Air Fryer Turkey Stuffed Peppers

Serving: 4 | Preparation Time: 30 minutes

Ingredients:

• 5 oz (150g) bell peppers (any color)
• 15 oz (450g) ground turkey
• 2 oz (60g) finely chopped onion
• 2 cloves garlic, minced
• 2.5 oz (75g) diced tomatoes
• 2 oz (60g) shredded cheddar cheese
• 1 oz (28g) almond flour

- 1 tsp dried oregano
- 1 tsp dried basil
- 1/2 tsp smoked paprika
- Salt and pepper to taste
- Cooking Spray

Instructions:

1. Preheat the air fryer to 350°F (177°C).
2. Cut off the tops of the bell peppers and remove the seeds and membranes.
3. In a bowl, mix together ground turkey, onion, garlic, diced tomatoes, cheddar cheese, almond flour, oregano, basil, smoked paprika, salt and pepper.
4. Stuff the peppers with the turkey mixture and place them in the air fryer basket.
5. Spray the peppers with cooking spray and cook for 20-25 minutes or until the peppers are tender and the turkey is cooked through.
6. Serve hot.

Nutritional values:
Calories: 259kcal | Fat: 13g | Protein: 24g | Carbs: 13g | Net carbs: 8g | Fiber: 5g | Cholesterol: 81mg | Sodium: 225mg | Potassium: 863mg

Air Fryer Turkey Slices with Balsamic Glaze

Serving: 4 | Preparation Time: 15 minutes

Ingredients:

- 15 oz (450g) turkey cutlets
- 2 oz (60ml) balsamic vinegar
- 1 tbsp olive oil
- 1 tsp honey
- 2 cloves garlic, minced
- Salt and pepper to taste
- Cooking spray

Instructions:

1. Preheat the air fryer to 375°F (190°C).
2. In a small bowl, whisk together balsamic vinegar, olive oil, honey, garlic, salt, and pepper to make the glaze.
3. Brush the turkey cutlets with the glaze on both sides.

4. Spray the air fryer basket with cooking spray and place the turkey cutlets in the basket.
5. Cook for 8-10 minutes or until the turkey is cooked through and golden brown, flipping halfway through and brushing with more glaze.
6. Serve hot, drizzled with any remaining glaze.

Note: Don't use excess honey or sugar in the recipe, so it will not increase your sugar level.

Nutritional values:
Calories: 172kcal | Fat: 4g | Protein: 25g | Carbs: 6g | Net carbs: 6g | Fiber: 0g | Cholesterol: 63mg | Sodium: 68mg | Potassium: 344mg

Chicken Recipes

Air Fryer Chicken Wings with Garlic-Parmesan Sauce

Serving: 4 | Preparation Time: 25 minutes

Ingredients:

- 30 oz (900g) chicken wings
- 1 tbsp olive oil
- 1/2 tsp garlic powder
- 1 oz (30g) grated parmesan cheese
- 2 tbsp butter, melted
- 2 cloves garlic, minced
- 1 tbsp chopped fresh parsley
- 1 tbsp lemon juice
- Cooking Spray
- Salt and pepper to taste

Instructions:

1. Preheat the air fryer to 380°F (193°C).
2. In a large bowl, toss chicken wings with olive oil, garlic powder, salt, and pepper until well coated.
3. Spray the air fryer basket with cooking spray and arrange the chicken wings in a single layer.
4. Cook for 20-25 minutes, flipping halfway through until golden brown and cooked through.
5. In a small bowl, whisk together parmesan cheese, melted butter, garlic, lemon juice, and parsley to make the garlic-parmesan sauce.
6. Toss the cooked chicken wings with the garlic-parmesan sauce until well coated.
7. Serve hot, garnished with more chopped parsley if desired.

Nutritional values:

Calories: 369kcal | Fat: 28g | Protein: 27g | Carbs: 2g | Net carbs: 2g | Fiber: 0g | Cholesterol: 146mg | Sodium: 494mg | Potassium: 259mg

Air Fryer Chicken Breasts with Lemon and Herb Marinade

Serving: 4 | Preparation Time: 35 minutes (including marinating time)

Ingredients:

- 15 oz (450g) skinless chicken breasts
- 2 tbsp olive oil
- 2 tbsp fresh lemon juice
- 2 cloves garlic, minced
- 1 tsp dried oregano
- 1 tsp dried thyme
- Cooking Spray
- Salt and pepper to taste

Instructions:

1. Preheat the air fryer to 375°F (190°C).
2. In a small bowl, whisk together olive oil, lemon juice, garlic, oregano, thyme, salt, and pepper to make the marinade.
3. Place chicken breasts in a shallow dish and pour the marinade over them, turning to coat well. Cover and refrigerate for at least 30 minutes or up to 4 hours.
4. Spray the air fryer basket with cooking spray and arrange the chicken breasts in a single layer.
5. Cook for 15-20 minutes, flipping halfway through, until the internal temperature of the chicken reaches 165°F (74°C).
6. Let the chicken rest for 5 minutes before slicing and serving.

Nutritional values:

Calories: 235kcal | Fat: 10g | Protein: 34g | Carbs: 2g | Net carbs: 2g | Fiber: 0g | Cholesterol: 98mg | Sodium: 148mg | Potassium: 561mg

Air Fryer Chicken Thighs with BBQ Rub

Serving: 4 | Preparation Time: 30 minutes

Ingredients:

- 7 oz (200g) bone-in, skin-on chicken thighs
- 2 tbsp olive oil
- 1 tsp honey
- 1 tbsp smoked paprika
- 1 tbsp chili powder
- 1 tsp garlic powder

- 1 tsp onion powder
- Cooking Spray
- Salt and pepper to taste

Instructions:

1. Preheat the air fryer to 375°F (190°C).
2. In a small bowl, whisk together honey, smoked paprika, chili powder, garlic powder, onion powder, salt, and pepper to make the BBQ rub.
3. Rub the chicken thighs with olive oil and sprinkle the BBQ rub on both sides, rubbing it in to ensure it adheres well.
4. Spray the air fryer basket with cooking spray and place the chicken thighs in a single layer.
5. Cook for 20-25 minutes, flipping halfway through, until the internal temperature of the chicken reaches 165°F (74°C).
6. If desired, brush the chicken thighs with BBQ sauce in the last 5 minutes of cooking.
7. Let the chicken rest for 5 minutes before serving.

Note: Don't use excess honey or sugar in the recipe, so it will not increase your sugar level.

Nutritional values:
Calories: 278kcal | Fat: 21g | Protein: 19g | Carbs: 5g | Net carbs: 4g | Fiber: 1g | Cholesterol: 110mg | Sodium: 298mg | Potassium: 274mg

Air Fryer Chicken Fajitas

Serving: 4 | Preparation Time: 25 minutes

Ingredients:

- 15 oz (450g) boneless, skinless chicken breasts, sliced into thin strips
- 4 oz (120g) red bell pepper, sliced
- 4 oz (120g) green bell pepper, sliced
- 2 oz (60g) yellow onion, sliced
- 2 tbsp olive oil
- 1 tbsp lime juice
- 2 cloves garlic, minced
- 1 tsp chili powder
- Cooking Spray
- Salt and pepper to taste

Instructions:

1. Preheat the air fryer to 375°F (190°C).

2. In a large bowl, whisk together olive oil, lime juice, garlic, chili powder, salt, and pepper.
3. Add chicken strips, bell peppers, and onion to the bowl and toss until coated evenly.
4. Spray the air fryer basket with cooking spray and add the chicken and vegetables in a single layer.
5. Cook for 15-20 minutes, flipping halfway through, until the chicken is cooked through and the vegetables are tender.
6. Serve with low-carb tortillas, if desired.

Nutritional values:
Calories: 245kcal | Fat: 11g | Protein: 27g | Carbs: 9g | Net carbs: 7g | Fiber: 2g | Cholesterol: 73mg | Sodium: 205mg | Potassium: 614mg

Air Fryer Chicken Satay Skewers

Serving: 4 | Preparation Time: 45 minutes (including marinating time)

Ingredients:

- 15 oz (450g) boneless, skinless chicken thighs cut into small cubes
- 2 oz (60ml) coconut milk
- 1 tbsp less sodium soy sauce
- 1 tbsp sesam oil
- 1 tbsp lime juice
- 1 tsp honey
- 1 tsp curry powder
- 1/2 tsp turmeric
- Cooking Spray
- Salt and pepper to taste
- Skewers

Instructions:

1. Preheat the air fryer to 375°F (190°C).
2. In a large bowl, whisk together coconut milk, soy sauce, sesam oil, lime juice, honey, curry powder, turmeric, salt, and pepper.
3. Add chicken cubes to the bowl and toss until coated evenly. Cover and marinate in the refrigerator for at least 30 minutes.
4. Thread the chicken onto skewers.
5. Spray the air fryer basket with cooking spray and add the skewers in a single layer.

6. Cook for 10-12 minutes, flipping halfway through, until the chicken is cooked through and slightly charred.

7. Serve with low-carb peanut sauce and sliced cucumber, if desired.

Note: Don't use excess honey or sugar in the recipe, so it will not increase your sugar level.

Nutritional values:

Calories: 280kcal | Fat: 16g | Protein: 30g | Carbs: 4g | Net carbs: 3g | Fiber: 1g | Cholesterol: 166mg | Sodium: 513mg | Potassium: 475mg

Air Fryer Chicken Parmesan

Serving: 4 | Preparation Time: 25 minutes

Ingredients:

• 7 oz (200g) boneless, skinless chicken breasts
• 1.88 oz (50g) almond flour
• 0.88 oz (25g) grated Parmesan cheese
• 1 tsp garlic powder
• 1 tsp dried oregano
• 1 tsp dried basil
• 1/2 tsp salt
• 1/4 tsp black pepper
• 1 egg, beaten
• 2 oz (60ml) tomato sauce
• 1.88 oz (50g) shredded mozzarella cheese

Instructions:

1. Preheat the air fryer to 390°F (200°C).

2. In a shallow bowl, mix almond flour, Parmesan cheese, garlic powder, dried oregano, dried basil, salt, and black pepper.

3. Dip chicken breasts into the beaten egg, then coat with the almond flour mixture.

4. Place the chicken in the air fryer basket in a single layer.

5. Air fry for 8-10 minutes on one side, then flip and air fry for an additional 4-6 minutes or until the chicken is cooked through and crispy.

6. Spoon tomato sauce over the chicken and sprinkle with shredded mozzarella cheese.

7. Air fry for another 2-3 minutes or until the cheese is melted and bubbly.

8. Serve hot with a side of zucchini noodles or your favorite low-carb pasta alternative.

Nutritional values:

Calories: 295kcal | Fat: 14g | Protein: 38g | Carbs: 5g | Net carbs: 3g | Fiber: 2g | Cholesterol: 173mg | Sodium: 609mg | Potassium: 418mg

Air Fryer Chicken Tenders with Spicy Dipping Sauce

Serving: 4 | Preparation Time: 20 minutes

Ingredients:

For the chicken tenders:

• 15 oz (450g) boneless, skinless chicken breasts cut into strips
• 0.88 oz (50g) almond flour
• 1/2 tsp paprika
• 1/2 tsp garlic powder
• 1/2 tsp salt
• 1/4 tsp black pepper
• 1 egg, beaten

For the spicy dipping sauce:

• 4 oz (120 g) low fat Greek yougurt
• 1 tbsp hot sauce
• 1 tsp honey
• 1/2 tsp garlic powder
• Cooking Spray

Instructions:

1. Preheat the air fryer to 400°F (200°C).

2. In a shallow bowl, mix almond flour, paprika, garlic powder, salt, and black pepper.

3. Dip chicken strips into the beaten egg, then coat with the almond flour mixture.

4. Spray the air fryer basket with cooking spray.

5. Place the chicken strips in the air fryer basket in a single layer, leaving space between each strip.

6. Air fry for 10-12 minutes, flipping once, or until the chicken is cooked through and crispy.

7. While the chicken is cooking, prepare the spicy dipping sauce by whisking together low fat Greek yougurt, hot sauce, honey, garlic powder, salt, and pepper in a small bowl.

8. Serve the chicken tenders hot with the spicy dipping sauce on the side.

Note: Don't use excess honey or sugar in the recipe, so it will not increase your sugar level.

Nutritional values:

Calories: 388kcal | Fat: 31g | Protein: 21g | Carbs: 7g | Net carbs: 6g | Fiber: 1g | Cholesterol: 133mg | Sodium: 883mg | Potassium: 339mg

Air Fryer Chicken Drumsticks with Ranch Seasoning

Serving: 4 | Preparation Time: 25 minutes

Ingredients:

• 5 oz (150g) chicken drumsticks
• 2 tbsp olive oil
• 1 tbsp ranch seasoning mix
• Salt and pepper to taste

Instructions:

1. Preheat the air fryer to 375°F (190°C).
2. In a small bowl, mix together the olive oil, salt, pepper and ranch seasoning.
3. Pat the chicken drumsticks dry with a paper towel, then brush them with the seasoned olive oil mixture.
4. Place the drumsticks in a single layer in the air fryer basket.
5. Cook for 20-25 minutes, flipping the drumsticks halfway through cooking, until the chicken is cooked through and the skin is crispy and golden brown.
6. Season with salt and pepper to taste before serving.

Nutritional values:

Calories: 320kcal | Fat: 22g | Protein: 28g | Carbs: 0g | Net carbs: 0g | Fiber: 0g | Cholesterol: 140mg | Sodium: 250mg | Potassium: 310mg

Air Fryer Chicken Teriyaki

Serving: 4 | Preparation time: 28 minutes

Ingredients:

• 7 oz (200g) boneless, skinless chicken breasts
• 4 oz (120ml) low-sodium soy sauce
• 1 oz (30ml) honey
• 2 oz (60ml) rice vinegar
• 2 garlic cloves, minced
• 1 tsp fresh ginger, grated
• 1 tbsp wholewheat flour
• 0.5 oz (15ml) Water

Instructions:

1. Preheat the air fryer to 400°F (200°C).
2. In a small bowl, whisk together the soy sauce, honey, rice vinegar, minced garlic, and grated ginger until well combined.
3. Pour half of the sauce mixture over the chicken breasts and let them marinate for 10 minutes.
4. In another small bowl, mix together the wholewheat flour and water until the wholewheat flour is dissolved.
5. Add the wholewheat flour mixture to the remaining sauce mixture and stir well.
6. Place the chicken breasts in the air fryer basket and discard the marinade.
7. Cook for 10 minutes, then flip the chicken breasts over and cook for another 10 minutes.
8. Brush the chicken breasts with the sauce mixture and cook for an additional 2-3 minutes.
9. Garnish with sesame seeds and chopped scallions (optional) and serve.

Note: Don't use excess honey or sugar in the recipe, so it will not increase your sugar level.

Nutritional values:

Calories: 276 kcal | Fat: 3g | Protein: 42g | Carbs: 18g | Net carbs: 16g | Fiber: 2g | Cholesterol: 110mg | Sodium: 1060mg | Potassium: 680mg

Air Fryer Chicken Souvlaki

Serving: 4 | Preparation time: 35 minutes

Ingredients:

• 7 oz (200g) boneless, skinless chicken breasts cut into 1-inch cubes
• 2 oz (60ml) olive oil
• 2 oz (60ml) lemon juice
• 1 tbsp red wine vinegar
• 2 garlic cloves, minced
• 1 tsp dried oregano
• 1 tsp salt
• 1/2 tsp black pepper
• Wooden skewers, soaked in water for at least 30 minutes

Instructions:

1. Preheat the air fryer to 400°F (200°C).

2. In a large bowl, whisk together the olive oil, lemon juice, red wine vinegar, minced garlic, dried oregano, salt, and black pepper until well combined.

3. Add the chicken cubes to the bowl and toss to coat evenly with the marinade.

4. Thread the chicken cubes onto the wooden skewers.

5. Place the skewers in the air fryer basket, leaving some space between them.

6. Cook for 8-10 minutes, then flip the skewers over and cook for another 8-10 minutes, until the chicken is cooked through and the juices run clear.

7. Serve and enjoy.

Nutritional values:
Calories: 245 kcal | Fat: 14g | Protein: 27g | Carbs: 2g | Net carbs: 2g | Fiber: 0g | Cholesterol: 85mg | Sodium: 380mg | Potassium: 463mg

Air Fryer Chicken Shawarma

Serving: 4 | Preparation time: 15 minutes | Cooking time: 25 minutes

Ingredients:

• 7 oz (200g) boneless, skinless chicken breasts, sliced into thin strips
• 2 oz (60ml) olive oil
• 2 tbsp lemon juice
• 2 garlic cloves, minced
• 1 tsp ground cumin
• 1 tsp paprika
• 1/2 tsp ground coriander
• 1/2 tsp ground cinnamon
• 1/4 tsp cayenne pepper
• Salt and black pepper, to taste
• Pita bread, lettuce, tomatoes, red onions, and tahini sauce for serving

Instructions:

1. Preheat the air fryer to 380°F (193°C).

2. In a large bowl, whisk together the olive oil, lemon juice, minced garlic, ground cumin, paprika, ground coriander, ground cinnamon, cayenne pepper, salt, and black pepper until well combined.

3. Add the chicken strips to the bowl and toss to coat evenly with the marinade.

4. Place the chicken in the air fryer basket in a single layer, leaving some space between the strips.

5. Cook for 10-12 minutes, then flip the chicken over and cook for another 10-12 minutes, until the chicken is cooked through and browned on both sides.

6. Serve the chicken shawarma in pita bread with lettuce, tomatoes and red onions.

Nutritional values:
Calories: 316 kcal | Fat: 15g | Protein: 29g | Carbs: 17g | Net carbs: 15g | Fiber: 2g | Cholesterol: 73mg | Sodium: 479mg | Potassium: 487mg

Air Fryer Chicken Nuggets

Serving: 4 | Preparation Time: 20 Minutes

Ingredients:

• 15 oz (450g) boneless, skinless chicken breasts cut into small pieces
• 2 oz (60g) whole wheat flour
• 1 tsp paprika
• 1 tsp garlic powder
• 1 tsp onion powder
• 1/2 tsp salt
• 1 large egg, beaten
• 4 oz (100g) panko low-carb breadcrumbs
• Cooking Spray

Instructions:

1. Preheat the air fryer to 400°F (200°C).

2. In a shallow bowl, mix together the flour, paprika, garlic powder, onion powder, salt.

3. In another shallow bowl, beat the egg.

4. In a third shallow bowl, add the panko low-carb breadcrumbs.

5. Coat each chicken piece with the flour mixture, then dip in the beaten egg, and finally coat with the panko breadcrumbs.

6. Place the chicken nuggets in a single layer in the air fryer basket.

7. Spray the chicken nuggets with cooking spray.

8. Cook for 8-10 minutes, flipping halfway through, or until the chicken is cooked through and the coating is golden brown and crispy.

9. Serve immediately with your favorite dipping sauce.

Nutritional values:
Calories: 250kcal | Fat: 6g | Protein: 29g | Carbs: 19g | Net carbs: 17g | Fiber: 2g | Cholesterol: 145mg | Sodium: 460mg | Potassium: 450mg

Air Fryer Chicken Quesadillas

Serving: 4 | Preparation Time: 20 Minutes

Ingredients:

• 9 oz (280g) cooked; shredded chicken
• 2 oz (60g) chopped onion
• 2.5 oz (75g) chopped bell pepper
• 1 tsp cumin
• 1 tsp chili powder
• 1/2 tsp salt
• 8.5 oz (240g) whole wheat tortillas (8-inch)
• 4 oz (100g) shredded cheddar cheese
• Salsa, sour cream, and guacamole for serving

Instructions:

1. Preheat the air fryer to 375°F (190°C).

2. In a large bowl, mix together the shredded chicken, chopped onion, chopped bell pepper, cumin, chili powder, and salt.

3. Place one tortilla on a flat surface and sprinkle 4 oz of the shredded cheese on one half of the tortilla.

4. Spoon 1/4 of the chicken mixture on top of the cheese.

5. Fold the other half of the tortilla over the chicken and cheese to create a half-circle.

6. Repeat with the remaining tortillas, cheese, and chicken mixture.

7. Place the quesadillas in the air fryer basket in a single layer.

8. Cook for 5-6 minutes, flipping halfway through, or until the tortillas are crispy and the cheese is melted.

9. Serve immediately with salsa, sour cream, and guacamole on the side.

Nutritional values:
Calories: 400kcal | Fat: 19g | Protein: 32g | Carbs: 26g | Net carbs: 22g | Fiber: 4g | Cholesterol: 90mg | Sodium: 900mg | Potassium: 430mg

Air Fryer Chicken Enchiladas

Serving: 4 | Preparation Time: 20 minutes

Ingredients:

• 15 oz (450g) cooked chicken, shredded (rotisserie or cooked chicken breast)
• 1 tbsp olive oil
• 1 oz (30g) onion, diced
• 14 oz (400g) less sodium enchilada sauce
• 1 tsp ground cumin
• Salt and pepper to taste
• 4 oz (120ml) low carb tortillas
• 4 oz (120g) shredded Mexican cheese blend
• Cooking Spray

Instructions:

1. Preheat your air fryer to 375°F (190°C).

2. In a large skillet, heat the olive oil over medium heat. Add the diced onion and cook until it becomes translucent, about 2-3 minutes.

3. Add the shredded chicken to the skillet, along with the ground cumin, salt, and pepper. Mix everything together, ensuring the chicken is well coated with the spices.

4. Pour in half of the enchilada sauce and mix it with the chicken until combined.

5. Take a low-carb tortilla and spoon a portion of the chicken mixture onto it. Roll it up tightly and place it seam-side down on a plate or tray. Repeat this step with the remaining tortillas and chicken mixture.

6. Once all the enchiladas are rolled, lightly spray them with cooking spray to promote crispiness during air frying.

7. Arrange the enchiladas in the air fryer basket in a single layer. You may need to cook them in batches depending on the size of your air fryer.

8. Air fry the enchiladas at 375°F (190°C) for 8-10 minutes or until they are heated through and the tortillas turn crispy.

9. While the enchiladas are air frying, warm the remaining enchilada sauce in a small saucepan over low heat.

10. Once the enchiladas are ready, remove them from the air fryer and transfer them to serving plates.

11. Pour the warmed enchilada sauce over the enchiladas, and sprinkle the shredded Mexican cheese blend on top.

Nutritional values:

Calories: 230kcal | Fat: 7g | Protein: 23g | Carbs: 19g | Net carbs: 14g | Fiber: 5 g | Cholesterol: 55mg | Sodium: 540mg | Potassium: 390mg

Air Fryer Chicken Lettuce Wraps

Serving: 4 | Preparation Time: 20 Minutes

Ingredients:

- 15 oz (450g) ground chicken
- 1 oz (30g) onion, chopped
- 2 garlic cloves, minced
- 1 tbsp ginger, minced
- 1 tbsp less sodium soy sauce
- 1 tbsp rice vinegar
- 1 tbsp sesame oil
- 2 oz (60g) green onions, sliced
- 6 oz (180g) lettuce, washed and separated into leaves
- Salt and pepper to taste

Instructions:

1. Preheat the air fryer to 400°F (200°C).

2. In a large bowl, combine the ground chicken, onion, garlic, ginger, soy sauce, rice vinegar, sesame oil, salt, and pepper. Mix well.

3. Form the chicken mixture into small meatballs, about 1 inch in diameter.

4. Place the meatballs in the air fryer basket, leaving a little space between them.

5. Air fry the chicken meatballs for 10-12 minutes, or until cooked through and golden brown on the outside.

6. To serve, place a few lettuce leaves on a plate and top with the chicken meatballs. Garnish with sliced green onions.

Nutritional values:

Calories: 218kcal | Fat: 13g | Protein: 19g | Carbs: 5g | Net carbs: 4g | Fiber: 1 g | Cholesterol: 98mg | Sodium: 481mg | Potassium: 516mg.

Chapter 5. Pork Recipes

Air Fryer Pork Chops with Mustard Cream

Serving: 4 | Preparation time: 5 minutes | Cooking time: 18-20 minutes

Ingredients:

- 7 oz (210g) bone-in pork chops, about 1 inch thick
- 2 tbsp olive oil
- 1 tsp paprika
- 1 tsp garlic powder
- 1/2 tsp salt
- 1/4 tsp black pepper
- 2 oz (60ml) heavy cream
- 2 tbsp Dijon mustard
- 2 tbsp chopped fresh parsley, for garnish

Instructions:

1. Preheat the air fryer to 400°F (200°C).
2. Brush the pork chops with olive oil and season them with paprika, garlic powder, salt, and black pepper on both sides.
3. Place the pork chops in the air fryer basket and cook for 10 minutes on one side.
4. Flip the pork chops over and cook for another 8-10 minutes until the internal temperature reaches 145°F (63°C).
5. While the pork chops are cooking, prepare the mustard cream sauce by combining the heavy cream and Dijon mustard in a small bowl.
6. Once the pork chops are done, remove them from the air fryer basket and let them rest for 5 minutes.
7. Serve the pork chops with the mustard cream sauce drizzled on top and garnish with chopped fresh parsley.

Nutritional values:
Calories: 385 kcal | Fat: 29g | Protein: 26g | Carbs: 3g | Net carbs: 2g | Fiber: 1g | Cholesterol: 104mg | Sodium: 510mg | Potassium: 479mg

Sauce Air Fryer Garlic and Herb Pork Tenderloin

Serving: 4 | Preparation time: 10 minutes | Cooking time: 20-25 minutes

Ingredients:

- 15 oz (450g) pork tenderloin
- 2 tbsp olive oil
- 2 garlic cloves, minced
- 1 tbsp dried rosemary
- 1 tbsp dried thyme
- 1 tsp salt
- 1/2 tsp black pepper

Instructions:

1. Preheat the air fryer to 375°F (190°C).
2. In a small bowl, whisk together the olive oil, minced garlic, dried rosemary, dried thyme, salt, and black pepper.
3. Pat the pork tenderloin dry with paper towels and brush it all over with the herb and garlic mixture.
4. Place the pork tenderloin in the air fryer basket and cook for 20-25 minutes, flipping it over halfway through cooking, until the internal temperature reaches 145°F (63°C) on a meat thermometer.
5. Remove the pork tenderloin from the air fryer and let it rest for 5 minutes before slicing it and serving.

Nutritional values:
Calories: 230 kcal | Fat: 10g | Protein: 34g | Carbs: 1g | Net carbs: 1g | Fiber: 0g | Cholesterol: 105mg | Sodium: 610mg | Potassium: 620mg

Air Fryer Balsamic Glazed Pork Tenderloin

Serving: 4 | Preparation time: 10 minutes | Cooking time: 20-25 minutes

Ingredients:

- 15 oz (450g) pork tenderloin

- 2 oz (60 ml) balsamic vinegar
- 2 tsp honey
- 2 garlic cloves, minced
- 1 tsp dried oregano
- 1/2 tsp salt
- 1/4 tsp black pepper

Instructions:

1. Preheat the air fryer to 375°F (190°C).
2. In a small bowl, whisk together the balsamic vinegar, honey, minced garlic, dried oregano, salt, and black pepper.
3. Pat the pork tenderloin dry with paper towels and brush it all over with the balsamic glaze mixture.
4. Place the pork tenderloin in the air fryer basket and cook for 20-25 minutes, flipping it over halfway through cooking, until the internal temperature reaches 145°F (63°C) on a meat thermometer.
5. Remove the pork tenderloin from the air fryer and let it rest for 5 minutes before slicing it and serving.

Note: Don't use excess honey or sugar in the recipe, so it will not increase your sugar level.

Nutritional values:

Calories: 220 kcal | Fat: 5g | Protein: 33g | Carbs: 10g | Net carbs: 10g | Fiber: 0g | Cholesterol: 105mg | Sodium: 400mg | Potassium: 620mg

Air Fryer BBQ Pulled Pork

Serving: 4 | Preparation time: 10 minutes | Cooking time: 1 hour

Ingredients:

- 15 oz (450g) pork shoulder or pork butt
- 4 oz (120ml) no added sugar BBQ sauce
- 2 oz (60ml) apple cider vinegar
- 1 tsp honey
- 1 tsp garlic powder
- 1 tsp paprika
- 1/2 tsp salt
- 1/4 tsp black pepper
- 1 tsp onion powder

Instructions:

1. Preheat the air fryer to 360°F (180°C).

2. In a small bowl, whisk together the BBQ sauce, apple cider vinegar, honey, smoked paprika, garlic powder, onion powder, salt, and black pepper until well combined.
3. Rub the mixture all over the pork roast.
4. Place the pork roast in the air fryer basket and cook for 25 minutes.
5. Flip the pork roast over and cook for another 25 minutes.
6. Remove the pork roast from the air fryer and let it cool for a few minutes.
7. Shred the pork with two forks, discarding any excess fat.
8. Toss the shredded pork in the remaining BBQ sauce mixture until well coated.
9. Return the shredded pork to the air fryer basket and cook for an additional 5-10 minutes, until the pork is hot and slightly crispy.
10. Serve on buns with coleslaw and pickles.

Note: Too much brown sugar can affect your sugar level

Nutritional values:

Calories: 326 kcal | Fat: 15g | Protein: 30g | Carbs: 19g | Net carbs: 17g | Fiber: 2g | Cholesterol: 95mg | Sodium: 643mg | Potassium: 625mg

Air Fryer Cuban Mojo Pork Tenderloin

Serving: 4 | Preparation time: 1 hour and 15 minutes (including marinating time) | Cooking time: 15-20 minutes

Ingredients:

- 15 oz (450g) pork tenderloin
- 4 cloves garlic, minced
- 2 oz (60ml) orange juice
- 2 oz (60ml) lime juice
- 1 oz (30ml) olive oil
- 1 tsp dried oregano
- 1 tsp ground cumin
- Salt and pepper to taste

Instructions:

1. Preheat the air fryer to 400°F (200°C).

2. In a small bowl, whisk together the olive oil, orange juice, lime juice, minced garlic, ground cumin, dried oregano, salt, and black pepper until well combined.

3. Place the pork tenderloin in a large zip-top bag and pour the marinade over it. Seal the bag and massage the pork to coat it evenly with the marinade.

4. Marinate in the refrigerator for at least 1 hour, or up to 8 hours.

5. Remove the pork tenderloin from the marinade and discard the excess marinade.

6. Place the pork tenderloin in the air fryer basket and cook for 15-20 minutes, flipping it over halfway through cooking, until the internal temperature of the pork reaches 145°F (63°C).

7. Let the pork rest for 5 minutes before slicing it into 1/2-inch (1.25 cm) rounds.

8. Serve with rice, black beans, and sliced avocado.

Nutritional values:
Calories: 225 kcal | Fat: 11g | Protein: 27g | Carbs: 2g | Net carbs: 2g | Fiber: 0g | Cholesterol: 83mg | Sodium: 402mg | Potassium: 601mg

Air Fryer Rosemary and Lemon Pork Chops

Serving: 4 | Preparation time: 10 minutes | Cooking time: 20-22 minutes

Ingredients:
- 15 oz (450g) bone-in pork chops, about 3/4-inch thick of
- 2 oz (60ml) olive oil
- 1 oz (30ml) lemon juice
- 2 garlic cloves, minced
- 2 oz (60g) fresh rosemary, finely chopped
- 1 tsp salt
- 1/2 tsp black pepper
- Lemon wedges, for serving

Instructions:
1. Preheat the air fryer to 375°F (190°C).

2. In a small bowl, whisk together the olive oil, lemon juice, minced garlic, chopped rosemary, salt, and black pepper until well combined.

3. Brush the pork chops with the marinade on both sides, reserving some for later.

4. Place the pork chops in the air fryer basket, leaving some space between them.

5. Cook for 10-12 minutes, then flip the pork chops over and brush with the remaining marinade.

6. Cook for another 8-10 minutes, until the pork chops are browned and cooked through, with an internal temperature of 145°F (63°C).

7. Serve the pork chops with lemon wedges.

Nutritional values:
Calories: 309 kcal | Fat: 22g | Protein: 25g | Carbs: 2g | Net carbs: 2g | Fiber: 0g | Cholesterol: 73mg | Sodium: 618mg | Potassium: 428mg

Air Fryer Honey Mustard Pork Tenderloin

Serving: 4 | Preparation time: 5 minutes | Cooking time: 25-30 minutes

Ingredients:
- 15 oz (450g) pork tenderloin
- 1 oz (30 ml) Dijon mustard
- 1 tsp honey
- 1 tbsp olive oil
- 1 tsp garlic powder
- 1/2 tsp salt
- 1/4 tsp black pepper

Instructions:
1. Preheat the air fryer to 400°F (200°C).

2. In a small bowl, whisk together the Dijon mustard, honey, olive oil, garlic powder, salt, and black pepper.

3. Brush the pork tenderloin with the honey mustard mixture, making sure to coat all sides.

4. Place the pork tenderloin in the air fryer basket.

5. Cook for 12-15 minutes, then flip the tenderloin over and cook for another 12-15 minutes, until the internal temperature of the pork reaches 145°F (63°C).

6. Let the pork rest for 5 minutes before slicing and serving.

Note: Too much honey can affect your sugar level

Nutritional values:
Calories: 240 kcal | Fat: 8g | Protein: 32g | Carbs: 10g | Net carbs: 9g | Fiber: 1g | Cholesterol: 100mg | Sodium: 460mg | Potassium: 562mg

Air Fryer Korean BBQ Pork Belly

Serving: 4 | time: 10 minutes | Cooking time: 20-24 minutes

Ingredients:

- 15 oz (450g) pork belly, sliced into 1/4-inch-thick pieces
- 2 oz (60 ml) less sodium soy sauce
- 1 tsp honey
- 1 tbsp sesame oil
- 1 tbsp rice vinegar
- 1 tsp garlic powder
- 1 tsp onion powder
- 1 tsp ginger powder
- 1/4 tsp black pepper and salt
- 1 oz (30g) Green onion
- 0.5 oz (15g) Sesame seeds

Instructions:

1. Preheat the air fryer to 400°F (200°C).
2. In a large bowl, whisk together the soy sauce, honey, sesame oil, rice vinegar, garlic powder, onion powder, ginger powder, salt and black pepper.
3. Add the sliced pork belly to the bowl and toss to coat evenly with the marinade.
4. Place the pork belly slices in the air fryer basket, leaving some space between them.
5. Cook for 10-12 minutes, then flip the pork belly over and cook for another 10-12 minutes, until the pork is cooked through and caramelized.
6. Serve with sliced green onions and sesame seeds.

Note: Too much honey and brown sugar can affect your sugar level

Nutritional values:
Calories: 400 kcal | Fat: 35g | Protein: 13g | Carbs: 10g | Net carbs: 9g | Fiber: 1g | Cholesterol: 52mg | Sodium: 1016mg | Potassium: 270mg

Air Fryer Pork Loin Roast with Garlic andHerbs

Serving: 4 | Preparation time: 10 minutes | Cooking time: 40-45 minutes

Ingredients:

- 30 oz (900g) pork loin roast
- 2 tbsp olive oil
- 2 garlic cloves, minced
- 0.4 oz (10g) fresh rosemary, chopped
- 1 tbsp fresh thyme, chopped
- 1 tsp salt
- 1/2 tsp black pepper

Instructions:

1. Preheat the air fryer to 360°F (180°C).
2. In a small bowl, mix together the olive oil, minced garlic, chopped rosemary, chopped thyme, salt, and black pepper.
3. Rub the herb mixture all over the pork loin roast.
4. Place the pork loin roast in the air fryer basket and cook for 20 minutes.
5. Flip the pork loin roast over and cook for another 20-25 minutes, or until the internal temperature reaches 145°F (63°C).
6. Let the pork loin roast rest for 5-10 minutes before slicing and serving.

Nutritional values:
Calories: 230 kcal | Fat: 13g | Protein: 25g | Carbs: 1g | Net carbs: 1g | Fiber: 0g | Cholesterol: 80mg | Sodium: 390mg | Potassium: 450mg

Air Fryer Pork Schnitzel

Serving: 4 | Preparation time: 15 minutes | Cooking time: 12 minutes

Ingredients:

- 15 oz (450g) boneless pork chops, pounded to 1/4-inch thickness
- 2 oz (60g) almond flour
- 2 eggs, beaten
- 4 oz (100g) panko low-carb breadcrumbs
- 1 tsp garlic powder
- 1 tsp onion powder
- 1/2 tsp paprika
- 1/2 tsp salt

- 1/4 tsp black pepper
- 1 tsp lemon juice
- Cooking spray

Instructions:

1. Preheat the air fryer to 400°F (200°C).
2. Place the flour in a shallow dish, the beaten eggs in another dish, and the panko breadcrumbs, garlic powder, onion powder, paprika, salt, and black pepper in a third dish.
3. Dip each pork chop in the flour, shaking off any excess. Then dip it into the egg mixture, coating it well. Finally, dip it in the breadcrumb mixture, pressing the breadcrumbs onto the pork chop to coat it thoroughly.
4. Spray the air fryer basket with cooking spray. Place the breaded pork chops in the basket, leaving some space between them.
5. Cook for 10-12 minutes, flipping them over halfway through the cooking time, until they are golden brown and crispy on the outside and cooked through on the inside.
6. Serve hot with a squeeze of lemon juice, a side salad, and your favorite dipping sauce.

Nutritional values:

Calories: 340 kcal | Fat: 12g | Protein: 36g | Carbs: 18g | Net carbs: 17g | Fiber: 1g | Cholesterol: 155mg | Sodium: 650mg | Potassium: 610mg

Air Fryer Teriyaki Pork Tenderloin

Serving: 4 | Preparation time: 15 minutes | Cooking time: 23 minutes

Ingredients:

- 15 oz (450g) pork tenderloin
- 2 oz (60ml) less sodium soy sauce
- 1 tsp honey
- 2 tbsp rice vinegar
- 1 tbsp sesame oil
- 2 cloves garlic, minced
- 1 tsp grated ginger
- Salt and pepper to taste
- Optional garnish: Sesame seeds and sliced green onions

Instructions:

1. Preheat your air fryer to 400°F (200°C) for about 5 minutes.
2. In a bowl, whisk together the soy sauce, honey, rice vinegar, sesame oil, minced garlic, salt, pepper and grated ginger to make the teriyaki marinade.
3. Place the pork tenderloin in a shallow dish or a resealable plastic bag. Pour the teriyaki marinade over the pork, making sure it is well coated. Allow the pork to marinate for at least 30 minutes or up to overnight in the refrigerator.
4. Remove the marinated pork from the dish or bag, reserving the marinade.
5. Place the pork tenderloin in the air fryer basket, making sure it's not overcrowded.
6. Cook the pork in the air fryer for about 20-25 minutes, or until the internal temperature reaches 145°F (63°C), flipping the tenderloin halfway through the cooking time.
7. While the pork is cooking, transfer the reserved marinade to a small saucepan. Bring it to a boil over medium heat and let it simmer for 5 minutes to thicken into a glaze.
8. Once the pork is cooked, remove it from the air fryer and let it rest for a few minutes before slicing.
9. Slice the pork tenderloin into medallions or desired thickness and drizzle the teriyaki glaze over the slices.
10. Garnish with sesame seeds and sliced green onions for added flavor and presentation.
11. Serve the Air Fryer Teriyaki Pork Tenderloin with steamed rice or your favorite side dishes, such as stir-fried vegetables or a fresh salad.

Note: Too much honey and brown sugar can affect your sugar level

Nutritional values:

Calories: 280 kcal | Fat: 3g | Protein: 32g | Carbs: 32g | Net carbs: 31g | Fiber: 1g | Cholesterol: 92mg | Sodium: 840mg | Potassium: 644mg

Air Fryer Pork Belly Burnt Ends

Serving: 4 | Preparation time: 10 minutes | Cooking time: 20-30 minutes

Ingredients:
- 15 oz (454g) pork belly
- 2 oz (60ml) BBQ sauce (look the sauce recipe in chapter 10)
- 2 tbsp unsalted butter
- 1 tbsp apple cider vinegar
- 1 tsp smoked paprika
- 1 tsp garlic powder
- 1 tsp onion powder
- 1/2 tsp salt and black pepper

Instructions:
1. Preheat the air fryer to 400°F (200°C).
2. Cut the pork belly into bite-size cubes and season with salt and black pepper.
3. In a small bowl, mix together the BBQ sauce, unsalted butter, apple cider vinegar, smoked paprika, garlic powder, onion powder.
4. Place the pork belly cubes in the air fryer basket and cook for 15-20 minutes or until crispy and browned.
5. After 10 minutes of cooking, remove the pork belly from the air fryer and toss in the BBQ sauce mixture.
6. Return the pork belly to the air fryer and continue cooking for an additional 5-10 minutes until the BBQ sauce has caramelized and the pork belly is fully cooked.
7. Remove from the air fryer and let them rest for a few minutes before serving.

Nutritional values:
Calories: 475 kcal | Fat: 42g | Protein: 13g | Carbs: 12g | Net carbs: 9g | Fiber: 3g | Cholesterol: 76mg | Sodium: 707mg | Potassium: 431mg

Air Fryer Cajun Pork Chops

Serving: 4 | Preparation time: 10 minutes | Cooking time: 12-15 minutes

Ingredients:
- 7 oz (200g) bone-in pork chops, about 1 inch thick
- 1 tbsp paprika
- 2 tsp garlic powder
- 1 tsp onion powder
- 1 tsp dried thyme
- 1 tsp dried oregano
- 1/2 tsp cayenne pepper
- 1/2 tsp salt
- 1/4 tsp black pepper
- 1 tbsp olive oil

Instructions:
1. Preheat the air fryer to 400°F (205°C).
2. In a small bowl, mix together the paprika, garlic powder, onion powder, dried thyme, dried oregano, cayenne pepper, salt, and black pepper.
3. Rub the spice mixture all over the pork chops.
4. Brush the pork chops with olive oil.
5. Place the pork chops in the air fryer basket, leaving some space between them.
6. Cook for 12-15 minutes or until the internal temperature reaches 145°F (63°C).
7. Flip the pork chops halfway through the cooking time.
8. Remove from the air fryer and let them rest for a few minutes before serving.

Nutritional values:
Calories: 295 kcal | Fat: 19g | Protein: 28g | Carbs: 3g | Net carbs: 2g | Fiber: 1g | Cholesterol: 89mg | Sodium: 466mg | Potassium: 568mg

Air Fryer Apple Cider Glazed Pork Tenderloin

Serving: 4 | Preparation time: 10 minutes | Cooking time: 15-20 minutes

Ingredients:
- 15 oz (450g) pork tenderloin
- 4 oz (120ml) apple cider
- 1 tbsp apple cider vinegar
- 1 tbsp olive oil
- 1 tsp honey
- 1 tsp ground cinnamon
- 1/2 tsp ground ginger
- 1/4 tsp ground nutmeg
- 1/4 tsp salt
- 1/4 tsp black pepper

Instructions:
1. Preheat the air fryer to 375°F (190°C).

2. In a small bowl, whisk together the apple cider, apple cider vinegar, olive oil, honey, ground cinnamon, ground ginger, ground nutmeg, salt, and black pepper.

3. Place the pork tenderloin in the air fryer basket.

4. Brush some of the apple cider glaze over the pork tenderloin.

5. Cook for 15-20 minutes or until the internal temperature reaches 145°F (63°C).

6. Baste the pork tenderloin with the remaining glaze halfway through the cooking time.

7. Remove from the air fryer and let it rest for a few minutes before slicing and serving.

Note: Too much brown sugar can affect your sugar level you have to control it.

Nutritional values:

Calories: 188 kcal | Fat: 5g | Protein: 28g | Carbs: 7g | Net carbs: 6g | Fiber: 1g | Cholesterol: 74mg | Sodium: 200mg | Potassium: 586mg

Air Fryer Sweet and Sour Pork Chops

Serving: 4 | Preparation time: 10 minutes | Cooking time: 12-15 minutes

Ingredients:

- 7 oz (200g) pork chops, bone-in
- 4 oz (120ml) ketchup (look the sauce recipe in chapter 10)
- 2 oz (60ml) apple cider vinegar
- 1.88 oz (50g) honey
- 1 tbsp less sodium soy sauce
- 1 tsp garlic powder
- 1/2 tsp onion powder
- Salt and pepper to taste

Instructions:

1. Preheat the air fryer to 375°F (190°C).

2. In a small bowl, whisk together the ketchup, apple cider vinegar, honey, soy sauce, garlic powder, onion powder, salt, and pepper.

3. Season the pork chops with salt and pepper on both sides.

4. Brush the sweet and sour sauce on both sides of the pork chops.

5. Place the pork chops in the air fryer basket.

6. Cook for 12-15 minutes or until the internal temperature reaches 145°F (63°C).

7. Flip the pork chops halfway through the cooking time and brush them with more sweet and sour sauce.

8. Serve hot with additional sweet and sour sauce on the side.

Note: Too much brown sugar can affect your sugar level you have to control it.

Nutritional values:

Calories: 357 kcal | Fat: 19g | Protein: 28g | Carbs: 18g | Net carbs: 16g | Fiber: 2g | Cholesterol: 89mg | Sodium: 750mg | Potassium: 563mg

Chapter 6.
Beef Recipes

Air Fryer Beef and Broccoli

Serving: 4 | Preparation time: 15 minutes | Cooking time: 15-20 minutes

Ingredients:

• 15 oz (450g) beef sirloin, sliced thinly
• 10 oz (300g) broccoli florets
• 2 oz (60g) red bell pepper, sliced
• 1 tbsp olive oil
• 2 tbsp less sodium soy sauce
• 1 tsp honey
• 1 tsp garlic powder
• 1/2 tsp ginger powder
• 1/4 tsp salt and black pepper

Instructions:

1. Preheat the air fryer to 375°F (190°C).
2. In a small bowl, mix together the olive oil, soy sauce, honey, garlic powder, ginger powder, salt and black pepper.
3. In a separate bowl, toss the beef slices with half of the soy sauce mixture.
4. Place the marinated beef in the air fryer basket, making sure it is not overcrowded.
5. Cook for 8-10 minutes or until the beef is browned and cooked through.
6. In a separate bowl, toss the broccoli florets and red bell pepper slices with the remaining soy sauce mixture.
7. Add the vegetables to the air fryer basket with the beef and cook for an additional 5-7 minutes or until the vegetables are tender.
8. Serve the beef and vegetables hot over rice or noodles.

Note: Too much honey and brown sugar can affect your sugar level you have to control it.

Nutritional values:

Calories: 296 kcal | Fat: 11g | Protein: 31g | Carbs: 17g | Net carbs: 14g | Fiber: 3g | Cholesterol: 69mg | Sodium: 775mg | Potassium: 754mg

Air Fryer Beef and Vegetable Kabobs

Serving: 4 | Preparation time: 15 minutes | Cooking time: 8-10 minutes

Ingredients:

• 15 oz (450g) beef sirloin, cut into 1-inch cubes
• 4 oz (120g) red bell pepper, seeded and cut into 1-inch pieces
• 4 oz (120g) green bell pepper, seeded and cut into 1-inch pieces
• 2 oz (60g) yellow onion, cut into 1-inch pieces
• 7 oz (200g) cherry tomatoes
• 1 tbsp olive oil
• 1 tsp garlic powder
• 1 tsp onion powder
• 1 tsp paprika
• 1/2 tsp salt
• 1/4 tsp black pepper
• Skewers

Instructions:

1. Preheat the air fryer to 400°F (205°C).
2. In a small bowl, mix together the olive oil, garlic powder, onion powder, paprika, salt, and black pepper.
3. Thread the beef, bell peppers, onion, and cherry tomatoes onto skewers.
4. Brush the kabobs with the olive oil and spice mixture.
5. Place the kabobs in the air fryer basket.
6. Cook for 8-10 minutes or until the beef is cooked to your liking, flipping the kabobs halfway through the cooking time.
7. Remove from the air fryer and let them rest for a few minutes before serving.

Nutritional values:

Calories: 285 kcal | Fat: 14g | Protein: 27g | Carbs: 11g | Net carbs: 8g | Fiber: 3g | Cholesterol: 69mg | Sodium: 471mg | Potassium: 830mg

Air Fryer Steak Fajitas

Serving: 4 | Preparation time: 15 minutes | Cooking time: 10-12 minutes

Ingredients:

- 15 oz (450g) flank steak, sliced into thin strips
- 4 oz (120g) red bell pepper, sliced into thin strips
- 4 oz (120g) green bell pepper, sliced into thin strips
- 2 oz (60g) yellow onion, sliced into thin strips
- 1 tbsp olive oil
- 1 tbsp chili powder
- 1/4 tsp salt and black pepper
- 7 oz (200g) low-carb tortillas

Instructions:

1. Preheat the air fryer to 400°F (200°C).
2. In a bowl, mix together the olive oil, salt, black pepper and chili powder.
3. Add the sliced steak, bell peppers, and onion to the bowl and toss to coat evenly.
4. Place the mixture in the air fryer basket, spreading it out in a single layer.
5. Cook for 10-12 minutes or until the steak is cooked through and the vegetables are tender, stirring halfway through the cooking time.
6. Warm the low-carb tortillas in the air fryer for 1-2 minutes, if desired.
7. Serve the steak and vegetables with the warmed tortillas.

Nutritional values:

Calories: 291 kcal | Fat: 11g | Protein: 28g | Carbs: 21g | Net carbs: 12g | Fiber: 9g | Cholesterol: 49mg | Sodium: 516mg | Potassium: 757mg

Air Fryer Beef Meatballs

Serving: 4 | Preparation time: 10 minutes | Cooking time: 10-12 minutes

Ingredients:

- 15 oz (450g) ground beef
- 1 oz (30g) almond flour
- 1 egg
- 1/2 tsp garlic powder
- 1/2 tsp onion powder
- 1/2 tsp salt
- 1/4 tsp black pepper

Instructions:

1. Preheat the air fryer to 375°F (190°C).
2. In a mixing bowl, combine ground beef, almond flour, egg, garlic powder, onion powder, salt, and black pepper. Mix until well combined.
3. Form the mixture into 12 evenly sized meatballs.
4. Place the meatballs in the air fryer basket, making sure they are not touching each other.
5. Cook for 10-12 minutes, flipping halfway through the cooking time.
6. Once cooked, remove from the air fryer and let them rest for a few minutes before serving.

Nutritional values:

Calories: 176 kcal | Fat: 12g | Protein: 16g | Carbs: 1g | Net carbs: 1g | Fiber: 0g | Cholesterol: 72mg | Sodium: 265mg | Potassium: 228mg

Air Fryer Beef and Mushroom Skewers

Serving: 4 | Preparation time: 15 minutes | Cooking time: 8-10 minutes

Ingredients:

- 15 oz (454g) beef sirloin, cut into 1-inch cubes
- 8 oz (227g) button mushrooms, cleaned and stems removed
- 1 tbsp olive oil
- 1 tbsp paprika
- 1 tsp garlic powder
- 1 tsp onion powder
- 1/2 tsp salt
- 1/4 tsp black pepper
- Skewers

Instructions:

1. Preheat the air fryer to 400°F (200°C).
2. In a large bowl, combine the beef cubes, cleaned mushrooms, olive oil, paprika, garlic powder, onion powder, salt, and black pepper. Toss well to coat evenly.
3. Thread the beef and mushrooms onto skewers, alternating between the two.
4. Place the skewers in the air fryer basket, leaving space between them to allow for even cooking.

5. Cook for 8-10 minutes, flipping the skewers half-way through, until the beef is cooked through to your desired doneness.

6. Serve hot and enjoy.

Nutritional values:

Calories: 250 kcal | Fat: 13g | Protein: 27g | Carbs: 6g | Net carbs: 4g | Fiber: 2g | Cholesterol: 74mg | Sodium: 368mg | Potassium: 772mg

Air Fryer Beef Stir Fry

Serving: 4 | Preparation time: 10 minutes | Cooking time: 10-12 minutes

Ingredients:

- 15 oz (450g) beef sirloin, thinly sliced
- 4 oz (120g) red bell pepper, sliced
- 4 oz (120g) green bell pepper, sliced
- 2 oz (60g) 1 onion, sliced
- 2 cloves garlic minced
- 2 tbsp less sodium soy sauce
- 1 tbsp rice vinegar
- 1 tbsp olive oil
- 1/2 tsp black pepper
- 1/2 tsp salt

Instructions:

1. Preheat the air fryer to 400°F (205°C).

2. In a small bowl, whisk together the soy sauce, rice vinegar, olive oil, minced garlic, salt, and black pepper.

3. In a large bowl, add the beef sirloin, sliced red and green bell peppers, and onion.

4. Pour the sauce over the beef and vegetables and toss to combine.

5. Add the beef and vegetable mixture to the air fryer basket and spread out in an even layer.

6. Cook for 10-12 minutes, stirring occasionally, or until the beef is cooked through and the vegetables are tender.

7. Serve hot over rice or with your favorite side dish.

Nutritional values:

Calories: 235 kcal | Fat: 10g | Protein: 29g | Carbs: 8g | Net carbs: 6g | Fiber: 2g | Cholesterol: 70mg | Sodium: 1049mg | Potassium: 540mg

Air Fryer Beef Brisket

Serving: 4 | Preparation time: 10 minutes | Cooking time: 30-40 minutes

Ingredients:

- 15 oz (454g) beef brisket
- 1 tbsp olive oil
- 1 tsp smoked paprika
- 1 tsp garlic powder
- 1 tsp onion powder
- 1/2 tsp salt
- 1/2 tsp black pepper

Instructions:

1. Preheat the air fryer to 375°F (190°C).

2. In a small bowl, mix together the olive oil, smoked paprika, garlic powder, onion powder, salt, and black pepper.

3. Pat the beef brisket dry with paper towels.

4. Brush the beef brisket on all sides with the spice mixture.

5. Place the beef brisket in the air fryer basket.

6. Cook for 30-40 minutes or until the internal temperature reaches 145°F (63°C) for medium-rare or 160°F (71°C) for medium.

7. Remove from the air fryer and let it rest for a few minutes before slicing.

Nutritional values:

Calories: 472 kcal | Fat: 35g | Protein: 35g | Carbs: 1g | Net carbs: 1g | Fiber: 0g | Cholesterol: 121mg | Sodium: 581mg | Potassium: 521mg

Air Fryer BBQ Beef Ribs

Serving: 4 | Preparation time: 10 minutes | Cooking time: 25-30 minutes

Ingredients:

- 30 oz (900g) beef ribs
- 4 oz (120ml) barbecue sauce (look the sauce recipe in chapter 10)
- 1 tbsp Worcestershire sauce (make sure it's sugar-free)
- 1 tsp garlic powder
- 1 tsp onion powder
- 1/2 tsp smoked paprika
- 1/2 tsp chili powder

- Salt and pepper to taste

Instructions:

1. Preheat the air fryer to 400°F (200°C).
2. In a small bowl, mix together the barbecue sauce, Worcestershire sauce, garlic powder, onion powder, smoked paprika, chili powder, salt, and pepper.
3. Rub the sauce mixture onto the beef ribs, ensuring they are evenly coated.
4. Place the ribs in the air fryer basket in a single layer.
5. Cook for 20-25 minutes, flipping the ribs halfway through cooking, until they are cooked through and the sauce is caramelized.
6. Remove from the air fryer and let them rest for a few minutes before serving.
7. Serve hot with additional barbecue sauce, if desired.

Note: Cooking times may vary depending on the thickness of the beef ribs. Adjust the cooking time accordingly to ensure they are cooked to your desired level of doneness.

Nutritional values per serving:
Calories: 450 kcal | Fat: 27g | Protein: 33g | Carbs: 19g | Net carbs: 15g | Fiber: 4g | Cholesterol: 115mg | Sodium: 590mg | Potassium: 760mg

Air Fryer Beef Satay with Peanut Sauce

Serving: 4 | Preparation time: 1 hour and 10 minutes (including marinating time) Cooking time: 8-10 minutes

Ingredients:
- 15 oz (450g) beef sirloin, cut into thin strips
- 2 oz (60ml) coconut milk
- 2 tbsp less sodium soy sauce
- 1 tbsp lime juice
- 2 tsp honey
- 1/2 tsp ground cumin
- 1/2 tsp ground coriander
- 1/4 tsp turmeric
- 1/4 tsp cayenne pepper
- Salt and pepper to taste
- 8 wooden skewers, soaked in water for 30 minutes

For the Peanut Sauce:
- 4 oz (125g) natural peanut butter
- 2 oz (60ml) coconut milk
- 2 tbsp less sodium soy sauce
- 1 tbsp lime juice
- 1 tsp honey
- 1/4 tsp cayenne pepper

Instructions:

1. In a bowl, mix together the coconut milk, soy sauce, lime juice, honey, cumin, coriander, turmeric, salt, pepper and cayenne pepper.
2. Add the beef strips to the marinade and stir to coat. Cover and refrigerate for at least 1 hour.
3. Preheat the air fryer to 400°F (200°C).
4. Thread the beef strips onto the skewers and place them in the air fryer basket.
5. Cook for 8-10 minutes, turning halfway through the cooking time, or until the beef is cooked to your liking.
6. While the beef is cooking, prepare the peanut sauce. In a small saucepan, combine the peanut butter, coconut milk, soy sauce, lime juice, honey, and cayenne pepper. Cook over low heat, stirring constantly, until the sauce is heated through and smooth.
7. Serve the beef satay with the peanut sauce on the side.

Note: Too much brown sugar can affect your sugar level, you have to control it.

Nutritional values:
Calories: 475 kcal | Fat: 33g | Protein: 31g | Carbs: 13g | Net carbs: 9g | Fiber: 4g | Cholesterol: 71mg | Sodium: 1190mg | Potassium: 662mg

Air Fryer Beef Kofta Kebabs

Serving: 4 | Preparation time: 15 minutes | Cooking time: 12-15 minutes

Ingredients:
- 15 oz (454g) ground beef
- 1 small onion, grated
- 0.5 oz (15g) chopped fresh parsley
- 2 cloves garlic, minced

- 1 tbsp ground cumin
- 1 tsp paprika
- 1/2 tsp salt
- 1/4 tsp black pepper

Instructions:

1. Preheat the air fryer to 375°F (190°C).
2. In a large bowl, mix together the ground beef, grated onion, chopped parsley, minced garlic, ground cumin, paprika, salt, and black pepper until well combined.
3. Form the mixture into 8-10 oblong shapes, about 3 inches long and 1 inch wide.
4. Place the kofta kebabs in the air fryer basket.
5. Cook for 12-15 minutes or until the internal temperature reaches 160°F (71°C), flipping them over halfway through the cooking time.
6. Serve with your favorite dipping sauce, salad, or pita bread.

Nutritional values:

Calories: 210 kcal | Fat: 16g | Protein: 15g | Carbs: 2g | Net carbs: 2g | Fiber: 0g | Cholesterol: 57mg | Sodium: 235mg | Potassium: 255mg

Lamb Recipes

Air Fryer Lamb Chops with Rosemary

Serving: 4 | Preparation time: 5 minutes | Cooking time: 10-12 minutes

Ingredients:

• 7 oz (200g) lamb chops, about 1 inch thick
• 1 tbsp olive oil
• 1 tbsp fresh rosemary leaves chopped
• 1 tsp salt
• 1/2 tsp black pepper

Instructions:

1. Preheat the air fryer to 400°F (200°C).
2. Rub the lamb chops on both sides with olive oil.
3. Sprinkle the fresh rosemary leaves, salt, and black pepper evenly over both sides of the lamb chops.
4. Place the lamb chops in the air fryer basket, making sure they are not touching each other.
5. Cook for 10-12 minutes for medium-rare, or until the internal temperature reaches 145°F (63°C).
6. Flip the lamb chops halfway through the cooking time.
7. Remove from the air fryer and let them rest for a few minutes before serving.

Nutritional values:

Calories: 225 kcal | Fat: 16g | Protein: 18g | Carbs: 0g | Net carbs: 0g | Fiber: 0g | Cholesterol: 70mg | Sodium: 620mg | Potassium: 240mg

Air Fryer Greek Lamb Meatballs

Serving: 4 | Preparation time: 15 minutes | Cooking time: 15 minutes

Ingredients:

• 15 oz (450g) ground lamb
• 0.8 oz (25g) almond flour
• 1 egg
• 2 tbsp olive oil
• 2 cloves garlic, minced
• 1 tbsp dried oregano
• 1 tsp salt
• 1/2 tsp black pepper
• Juice of 1/2 lemon
• 2 oz (60g) crumbled feta cheese
• Fresh parsley, chopped, for garnish

Instructions:

1. Preheat the air fryer to 375°F (190°C).
2. In a large bowl, combine the ground lamb, almond flour, egg, olive oil, minced garlic, dried oregano, salt, black pepper, and lemon juice. Mix well.
3. Roll the lamb mixture into 12 meatballs.
4. Place the meatballs in the air fryer basket.
5. Cook for 10-12 minutes, flipping the meatballs halfway through the cooking time.
6. Sprinkle the crumbled feta cheese over the meatballs.
7. Cook for an additional 2-3 minutes, or until the cheese is melted and bubbly.
8. Garnish with fresh parsley and serve.

Nutritional values:

Calories: 347 kcal | Fat: 29g | Protein: 19g | Carbs: 3g | Net carbs: 2g | Fiber: 1g | Cholesterol: 97mg | Sodium: 454mg | Potassium: 276mg

Air Fryer Lamb and Vegetable Skewers

Serving: 4 | Preparation time: 15 minutes | Cooking time: 15-20 minutes

Ingredients:

• 15 oz (450g) lamb shoulder, cut into 1-inch cubes
• 4 oz (120g) red bell pepper, seeded and cut into 1-inch pieces
• 4 oz (120g) yellow bell pepper, seeded and cut into 1-inch pieces
• 1 zucchini, cut into 1-inch pieces
• 2 oz (60g) red onion, cut into 1-inch pieces
• 2 tbsp olive oil
• 2 cloves garlic, minced

- 1 tsp salt
- 1/2 tsp black pepper
- Skewers

Instructions:

1. Preheat the air fryer to 375°F (190°C).
2. In a large bowl, mix together the olive oil, minced garlic, salt, and black pepper.
3. Add the lamb, bell peppers, zucchini, and red onion to the bowl and toss until the vegetables and lamb are evenly coated with the mixture.
4. Thread the lamb and vegetables onto skewers, alternating between the different ingredients.
5. Place the skewers in the air fryer basket.
6. Cook for 15-20 minutes or until the lamb is cooked through and the vegetables are tender, flipping the skewers halfway through the cooking time.
7. Remove from the air fryer and let the skewers rest for a few minutes before serving.

Nutritional values:

Calories: 338 kcal | Fat: 24g | Protein: 23g | Carbs: 10g | Net carbs: 8g | Fiber: 2g | Cholesterol: 76mg | Sodium: 650mg | Potassium: 540mg

Air Fryer Lamb and Chickpea Stew

Serving: 4 | Preparation time: 10 minutes | Cooking time: 30-35 minutes

Ingredients:

- 15 oz (450g) lamb stew meat, cut into bite-size pieces
- 2 oz (60g) chickpeas, drained and rinsed
- 1 oz (30g) onion, diced
- 2 cloves garlic, minced
- 1 tsp cumin
- 1 tsp smoked paprika
- 2 oz (60g) low-sodium chicken broth
- Salt and pepper to taste

Instructions:

1. Preheat the air fryer to 400°F (200°C).
2. In a large bowl, combine the lamb stew meat, chickpeas, onion, garlic, cumin, salt, pepper and smoked paprika.
3. Mix well to combine all the ingredients.

4. Pour the mixture into the air fryer basket and spread it out evenly.
5. Cook for 10 minutes.
6. Add the chicken broth to the basket and mix everything together.
7. Cook for another 15-20 minutes, or until the lamb is cooked through and the chickpeas are tender.
8. Serve hot and enjoy!

Nutritional values per serving:

Calories: 315kcal | Fat: 11g | Protein: 31g | Carbs: 23g | Net carbs: 17g | Fiber: 6g | Cholesterol: 87mg | Sodium: 347mg | Potassium: 688mgc

Air Fryer Lamb Shanks with Garlic and Herbs

Serving: 4 | Preparation time: 10 minutes | Cooking time: 30-35 minutes

Ingredients:

- 7 oz (200g) lamb shanks
- 4 cloves garlic, minced
- 1 tbsp olive oil
- 1 tsp dried rosemary
- 1 tsp dried thyme
- 1/2 tsp salt
- 1/4 tsp black pepper

Instructions:

1. Preheat the air fryer to 375°F (190°C).
2. In a small bowl, mix together the minced garlic, olive oil, dried rosemary, dried thyme, salt, and black pepper.
3. Pat the lamb shanks dry with paper towels.
4. Rub the garlic and herb mixture all over the lamb shanks.
5. Place the lamb shanks in the air fryer basket.
6. Cook for 30-35 minutes or until the internal temperature reaches 145°F (63°C) for medium-rare or 160°F (71°C) for medium.
7. Flip the lamb shanks halfway through the cooking time.
8. Let the lamb shanks rest for a few minutes before serving.

Nutritional values:

Calories: 534 kcal | Fat: 36g | Protein: 47g | Carbs: 1g | Net carbs: 1g | Fiber: 0g | Cholesterol: 205mg | Sodium: 439mg | Potassium: 725mg

Air Fryer Lamb Kofta Kebabs

Serving: 4 | Preparation time: 15 minutes | Cooking time: 10-12 minutes

Ingredients:

- 15 oz (450g) ground lamb
- 1 oz (30g) onion, grated
- 2 cloves garlic, minced
- 1 oz (25g) fresh parsley, chopped
- 1 tsp ground cumin
- 1 tsp ground coriander
- 1/2 tsp ground cinnamon
- 1/2 tsp ground allspice
- 1/2 tsp salt
- 1/4 tsp black pepper
- Skewer

Instructions:

1. Preheat the air fryer to 375°F (190°C).
2. In a large mixing bowl, combine the ground lamb, grated onion, minced garlic, chopped parsley, ground cumin, ground coriander, ground cinnamon, ground allspice, salt, and black pepper. Mix well until all ingredients are well combined.
3. Divide the mixture into 8 equal portions.
4. Take one portion and shape it into a sausage-shaped log around a skewer.
5. Repeat with the remaining portions, placing them onto skewers.
6. Place the skewers in the air fryer basket, making sure they don't touch each other.
7. Cook for 10-12 minutes or until the internal temperature of the lamb reaches 160°F (71°C).
8. Flip the skewers halfway through the cooking time.
9. Serve hot with your favorite dipping sauce or tzatziki.

Note: You can try adding some acidity to your dish with a squeeze of lemon juice or a splash of vinegar.

Nutritional values:

Calories: 216 kcal | Fat: 15g | Protein: 17g | Carbs: 2g | Net carbs: 2g | Fiber: 0g | Cholesterol: 65mg | Sodium: 271mg | Potassium: 246mg

Air Fryer Moroccan Spiced Lamb Chops

Serving: 4 | Preparation time: 10 minutes | Cooking time: 15 minutes

Ingredients:

- 8 oz (240g) lamb chops (approximately 1-inch thick)
- 2 tbsp olive oil
- 1 tsp ground cumin
- 1 tsp ground coriander
- 1 tsp paprika
- 1/2 tsp ground cinnamon
- 1/2 tsp ground ginger
- Salt and pepper to taste
- Fresh cilantro or parsley, for garnish

Instructions:

1. Preheat your air fryer to 400°F (200°C).
2. In a small bowl, mix together the ground cumin, ground coriander, paprika, ground cinnamon, ground ginger, salt, and pepper to create the spice rub.
3. Rub the spice mixture onto both sides of the lamb chops, ensuring they are well coated.
4. Brush each lamb chop with olive oil to promote browning and moisture.
5. Place the lamb chops in a single layer in the air fryer basket or tray.
6. Cook the lamb chops in the air fryer for 12-15 minutes, flipping them halfway through cooking, until they reach your desired level of doneness. For medium-rare, the internal temperature should be around 145°F (63°C).
7. Once cooked, remove the lamb chops from the air fryer and let them rest for a few minutes before serving.
8. Garnish with fresh cilantro or parsley.
9. Serve the Moroccan spiced lamb chops hot.

Nutritional values:
Calories: 280 kcal | Fat: 20g | Protein: 23g | Carbs: 1g | Net carbs: 1g | Fiber: 0g | Cholesterol: 85mg | Sodium: 70mg | Potassium: 320mg

Air Fryer Lamb Curry

Serving: 4 | Preparation time: 15 minutes | Cooking time: 10-12 minutes

Ingredients:

- 15 oz (450g) boneless lamb, cut into bite-sized pieces
- 1 oz (30g) onion, finely chopped
- 2 cloves garlic, minced
- 1 tbsp vegetable oil
- 2 tbsp curry powder
- 1 tsp ground cumin
- 1/2 tsp turmeric powder
- 4 oz (120ml) canned diced tomatoes
- 4 oz (120ml) coconut milk
- Salt and pepper to taste
- Fresh cilantro, for garnish

Instructions:

1. Preheat the air fryer to 375°F (190°C).
2. In a bowl, mix together the curry powder, ground cumin, and turmeric powder.
3. In the air fryer basket, add the lamb pieces and sprinkle them with half of the spice mixture. Toss to coat the lamb evenly.
4. Place the onion and garlic in the air fryer basket with the lamb.
5. Drizzle the vegetable oil over the ingredients in the basket and mix well.
6. Cook for 12-15 minutes, shaking the basket halfway through, until the lamb is browned and cooked to your desired level of doneness.
7. In a saucepan over medium heat, combine the canned diced tomatoes, coconut milk, and the remaining spice mixture. Stir well.
8. Add the cooked lamb, onion, and garlic from the air fryer basket to the saucepan. Season with salt and pepper to taste.
9. Simmer for 5-7 minutes to allow the flavors to meld together.
10. Garnish with fresh cilantro and serve hot with steamed rice or naan bread.

Nutritional values:
Calories: 320 kcal | Fat: 22g | Protein: 23g | Carbs: 8g | Net carbs: 6g | Fiber: 2g | Cholesterol: 70mg | Sodium: 180mg | Potassium: 610mg

Air Fryer Lamb and Eggplant

Servings: 4 | Preparation time: 10 minutes | Cooking time: 12-15 minutes

Ingredients:

- 15 oz (450g) lamb leg steak, cut into cubes
- 2 oz (60g) medium eggplant, cut into chunks
- 2 tbsp olive oil
- 1 tsp ground cumin
- 1 tsp ground coriander
- 1/2 tsp paprika
- 1/2 tsp garlic powder
- Salt and pepper to taste
- Fresh parsley, chopped (for garnish)

Instructions:

1. Preheat the air fryer to 400°F (200°C).
2. In a bowl, combine the cubed lamb, olive oil, ground cumin, ground coriander, paprika, garlic powder, salt, and pepper. Mix well to evenly coat the lamb.
3. Place the seasoned lamb and eggplant chunks in the air fryer basket.
4. Cook for 12-15 minutes, shaking the basket halfway through, or until the lamb is cooked to your desired doneness and the eggplant is tender and slightly charred.
5. Remove from the air fryer and let it rest for a few minutes.
6. Garnish with fresh chopped parsley before serving.

Note: If you want to add some extra flavor to this recipe, try adding some lemon juice or lemon zest to the lamb and eggplant mixture before cooking.

Nutritional values:
Calories: 280kcal | Fat: 18g | Protein: 24g | Carbs: 7g | Net carbs: 5g | Fiber: 2g | Cholesterol: 80mg | Sodium: 90mg | Potassium: 540mg

Air Fryer Lamb Burgers

Serving: 4 | Preparation time: 15 minutes | Cooking time: 10-12 minutes

Ingredients:

- 15 oz (450g) pound ground lamb
- 1 oz (30g) finely chopped onion
- 2 cloves garlic, minced
- 1 tbsp chopped fresh parsley
- 1 tsp ground cumin
- 1/2 tsp ground coriander
- 1/2 tsp salt
- 1/4 tsp black pepper
- 10 oz (300g) whole-wheat burger buns
- Lettuce, tomato, onion slices (for toppings)

Instructions:

1. In a mixing bowl, combine the ground lamb, chopped onion, minced garlic, parsley, cumin, coriander, salt, and black pepper. Mix well to evenly distribute the seasonings throughout the meat.

2. Divide the mixture into four equal portions and shape each portion into a patty.

3. Preheat the air fryer to 375°F (190°C).

4. Place the lamb patties in the air fryer basket in a single layer. Cook for 8-10 minutes, flipping the patties halfway through cooking, until they reach your desired level of doneness.

5. While the patties are cooking, lightly toast the burger buns.

6. Remove the lamb patties from the air fryer and assemble the burgers with your preferred toppings.

7. Serve hot.

Note: You can customize your lamb burgers by adding additional toppings and condiments of your choice. Enjoy your air fryer lamb burgers!

Nutritional values:

Calories: 320kcal | Fat: 20g | Protein: 22g | Carbs: 11g | Net carbs: 10g | Fiber: 1g | Cholesterol: 83mg | Sodium: 470mg

Chapter 7.
Fish Recipes

Air Fryer Lemon Garlic Salmon

Serving: 4 | Preparation time: 5 minutes | Cooking time: 8-10 minutes

Ingredients:

• 20 oz (600g) salmon fillets, skin on
• 2 tbsp olive oil
• 2 cloves garlic, minced
• 1 lemon, sliced
• Salt and pepper to taste
• Fresh parsley for garnish

Instructions:

1. Preheat the air fryer to 375°F (190°C).
2. Pat the salmon fillets dry and season with salt and pepper on both sides.
3. In a small bowl, mix together the olive oil and minced garlic.
4. Brush the salmon fillets with the garlic oil mixture.
5. Place the salmon fillets, skin side down, in the air fryer basket and top with lemon slices.
6. Air fry the salmon for 8-10 minutes, or until it is cooked through and flakes easily with a fork.
7. Garnish with fresh parsley before serving.

Nutritional values:

Calories: 319 kcal | Fat: 20g | Protein: 31g | Carbs: 3g | Net carbs: 3g | Fiber: 0g | Cholesterol: 77mg | Sodium: 65mg | Potassium: 832mg

Air Fryer Parmesan Crusted Tilapia

Serving: 4 | Preparation time: 10 minutes | Cooking time: 10-12 minutes

Ingredients:

• 20 oz (600g) tilapia fillets
• 2 oz (60g) almond flour
• 1 oz (25g) grated Parmesan cheese
• 1 tsp garlic powder
• 1 tsp dried basil
• 1/2 tsp paprika
• 1/2 tsp salt
• 1/4 tsp black pepper
• 2 tbsp olive oil

Instructions:

1. Preheat the air fryer to 400°F (200°C).
2. In a shallow dish, combine the almond flour, grated Parmesan cheese, garlic powder, dried basil, paprika, salt, and black pepper.
3. Dip the tilapia fillets into the mixture, making sure to coat them well on both sides.
4. Brush each fillet with olive oil.
5. Place the fillets in the air fryer basket, making sure they are not touching.
6. Air fry at 400°F (200°C) for 10-12 minutes, or until the crust is golden brown and the fish is cooked through.
7. Serve hot with your favorite side dish.

Nutritional values:

Calories: 326 kcal | Fat: 20g | Protein: 32g | Carbs: 6g | Net carbs: 4g | Fiber: 2g | Cholesterol: 83mg | Sodium: 598mg | Potassium: 511mg

Air Fryer Fish Tacos

Serving: 4 | Preparation time: 10 minutes Cooking time: 8-10 minutes

Ingredients:

• 15 oz (450g) firm white fish fillets, such as cod or tilapia
• 1 tbsp olive oil
• 1 tbsp taco seasoning
• 1 lime, cut into wedges
• 1 oz (30g) red onion, thinly sliced
• 8 oz (240g) low-carb tortillas
• 1 oz (30g) jalapeño pepper, seeded and thinly sliced
• Salt and pepper to taste

Instructions:

1. Preheat the air fryer to 375°F (190°C).
2. Season the fish fillets with salt, pepper, and taco seasoning.
3. Place the fish fillets in the air fryer basket and drizzle with olive oil.
4. Air fry the fish for 8-10 minutes, or until it is cooked through and flakes easily with a fork.
5. While the fish is cooking, warm the low-carb tortillas in the air fryer for 1-2 minutes.
6. Assemble the tacos by placing a piece of fish on each tortilla, and topping with red onion and jalapeño slices.
7. Squeeze a lime wedge over each taco before serving.

Nutritional values:
Calories: 247 kcal | Fat: 7g | Protein: 26g | Carbs: 20g | Net carbs: 17g | Fiber: 3g | Cholesterol: 51mg | Sodium: 311mg | Potassium: 469mg

Air Fryer Fish and Chips

Serving: 4 | Preparation time: 15 minutes | Cooking time: 8-10 minutes

Ingredients:

- 15 oz (450g) white fish fillets (such as cod, haddock, or tilapia)
- 2 oz (60g) whole wheat flour
- 1/4 tsp salt
- 1/4 tsp black pepper
- 4 oz (120g) panko low-carb breadcrumbs
- Cooking spray
- Lemon wedges, for serving

Instructions:

1. Preheat the air fryer to 390°F (200°C).
2. Cut the fish into strips or chunks.
3. In a shallow dish, mix together the flour, salt, and black pepper.
4. Place the panko breadcrumbs in another shallow dish.
5. Dip each piece of fish in the batter, allowing any excess batter to drip off, then coat it in the panko breadcrumbs, pressing lightly to make sure the coating sticks.

6. Place the fish in the air fryer basket, leaving some space between them to ensure they cook evenly.
7. Spray the fish with cooking spray to help them brown.
8. Air fry the fish for 8-10 minutes, flipping them halfway through, until they are golden brown and cooked through.
9. Serve hot with lemon wedges and your favorite dipping sauce.

Nutritional values:
Calories: 310 kcal | Fat: 6g | Protein: 29g | Carbs: 33g | Net carbs: 30g | Fiber: 3g | Cholesterol: 91mg | Sodium: 488mg | Potassium: 558mg

Air Fryer Cajun Salmon

Serving: 4 | Preparation time: 5 minutes | Cooking time: 8-10 minutes

Ingredients:

- 24 oz (780g) salmon fillets
- 2 tbsp olive oil
- 1 tbsp Cajun seasoning
- 1 lemon, sliced
- Salt and pepper to taste

Instructions:

1. Preheat the air fryer to 400°F (200°C).
2. Season the salmon fillets with salt, pepper, and cajun seasoning on both sides.
3. Drizzle the salmon fillets with olive oil.
4. Place the salmon fillets in the air fryer basket and top each fillet with a slice of lemon.
5. Air fry for 8-10 minutes, or until the salmon is cooked through and flakes easily with a fork.

Nutritional values:
Calories: 371 kcal | Fat: 22g | Protein: 37g | Carbs: 2g | Net carbs: 1g | Fiber: 1g | Cholesterol: 109mg | Sodium: 283mg | Potassium: 953mg

Air Fryer Blackened Catfish

Serving: 4 | Preparation time: 10 minutes | Cooking time: 8-10 minutes

Ingredients:

- 6 oz (170g) catfish fillets
- 2 tbsp olive oil

- 1 tbsp blackened seasoning
- 1 tsp paprika
- 1/2 tsp garlic powder
- 1/4 tsp cayenne pepper
- Salt and pepper to taste
- Lemon wedges

Instructions:

1. Preheat the air fryer to 400°F (205°C).
2. Mix together the blackened seasoning, paprika, garlic powder, cayenne pepper, salt, and pepper in a small bowl.
3. Brush the catfish fillets with olive oil and sprinkle the seasoning mixture over both sides of the fillets.
4. Place the catfish fillets in the air fryer basket and air fry for 8-10 minutes, or until the fish is cooked through and flakes easily with a fork.
5. Serve hot with lemon wedges and your favorite sides.

Nutritional values:

Calories: 284 kcal | Fat: 12g | Protein: 36g | Carbs: 1g | Net carbs: 1g | Fiber: 0g | Cholesterol: 109mg | Sodium: 435mg | Potassium: 579mg

Air Fryer Lemon Dill Cod

Serving: 4 | Preparation time: 25 minutes | Cooking time: 8-10 minutes

Ingredients:

- 4 oz (120g) cod fillets
- 2 oz (60ml) olive oil
- 1 tsp honey
- 2 cloves garlic, minced
- 1 tsp dried dill
- 1/2 tsp salt
- 1/4 tsp black pepper
- Lemon wedges, for serving
- 2 tsp freshly squeezed lemon juice

Instructions:

1. Preheat the air fryer to 375°F (190°C).
2. In a small mixing bowl, whisk together the olive oil, lemon juice, honey, minced garlic, dried dill, salt, and black pepper.

3. Place the cod fillets into a shallow dish and pour the marinade over them. Marinate for 15-20 minutes.
4. Remove the cod fillets from the marinade and place them onto the air fryer basket.
5. Cook for 8-10 minutes or until the internal temperature of the cod reaches 145°F (63°C).
6. Flip the fillets halfway through the cooking time.
7. Serve hot with lemon wedges.

Note: The use of too much sugar or honey might affect your sugar level, you have to control it.

Nutritional values:

Calories: 233 kcal | Fat: 13g | Protein: 24g | Carbs: 4g | Net carbs: 4g | Fiber: 0g | Cholesterol: 54mg | Sodium: 361mg | Potassium: 514mg

Air Fryer Crispy Fish Fillets

Serving: 4 | Preparation time: 10 minutes | Cooking time: 10-12 minutes

Ingredients:

- 4 oz (120g) fish fillets (such as cod, tilapia, or catfish)
- 1 oz (30g) almond flour
- 0.88 oz (20g) grated parmesan cheese
- 1/2 tsp garlic powder
- 1/4 tsp black pepper
- 1 large egg, beaten
- 1/2 tsp salt
- Cooking spray
- Lemon wedges, for serving

Instructions:

1. Preheat the air fryer to 400°F (200°C).
2. In a shallow bowl, mix together the almond flour, parmesan cheese, garlic powder, salt, and black pepper.
3. Dip each fish fillet into the beaten egg, then coat in the almond flour mixture.
4. Place the fish fillets onto the air fryer basket, making sure they are not touching each other.
5. Lightly spray the fish fillets with cooking spray.
6. Cook for 10-12 minutes or until the fish is golden brown and crispy and the internal temperature reaches 145°F (63°C).

7. Serve the fish fillets hot with lemon wedges and tartar sauce, if desired.

Nutritional values:

Calories: 277 kcal | Fat: 15g | Protein: 28g | Carbs: 5g | Net carbs: 3g | Fiber: 2g | Cholesterol: 126mg | Sodium: 543mg | Potassium: 438mg

Air Fryer Panko Crusted Fish Fillets

Serving 4 | Preparation time: 10 Minutes | Cooking Time: 10 Minutes

Ingredients:

• 4 oz (120g) fish fillets (such as cod, haddock, or tilapia)
• 2 oz (60g) wholewheat flour
• 2 eggs, beaten
• 1.88 oz (50g) panko low-carb breadcrumbs
• 1/2 tsp garlic powder
• 1/2 tsp onion powder
• 1/2 tsp paprika
• 1/4 tsp salt
• Cooking spray
• Lemon wedges, for serving

Instructions:

1. Preheat the air fryer to 400°F (200°C).
2. Place the flour in a shallow bowl.
3. In another shallow bowl, beat the eggs.
4. In a third shallow bowl, combine the panko breadcrumbs, garlic powder, onion powder, paprika, and salt.
5. Dredge each fish fillet in the flour, shaking off any excess.
6. Dip each fish fillet in the beaten eggs, making sure it is fully coated.
7. Press each fish fillet into the panko mixture, making sure it is fully coated.
8. Place the fish fillets in the air fryer basket, making sure they are not touching each other.
9. Spray the fish fillets with cooking spray.
10. Cook for 8-10 minutes or until the fish is cooked through and the coating is crispy.
11. Serve the Panko Crusted Fish Fillets hot with lemon wedges and tartar sauce, if desired.

Nutritional values:

Calories: 291 kcal | Fat: 9g | Protein: 31g | Carbs: 21g | Net carbs: 19g | Fiber: 2g | Cholesterol: 148mg | Sodium: 449mg

Air Fryer Herb Crusted Trout

Serving: 4 | Preparation Time: 20 minutes

Ingredients:

• 24 oz (720g) trout fillets
• 2 tbsp olive oil
• 1 oz (25 g) almond flour
• 2 tbsp chopped fresh parsley
• 1 tbsp chopped fresh dill
• 1 tbsp chopped fresh thyme
• 1 tsp lemon zest
• Salt and pepper to taste
• Cooking spray
• Lemon wedges, for serving

Instructions:

1. Preheat the air fryer to 375°F (190°C).
2. In a shallow bowl, combine almond flour, chopped parsley, chopped dill, chopped thyme, lemon zest, salt, and pepper.
3. Brush both sides of the trout fillets with olive oil.
4. Dredge the trout fillets in the herb mixture, pressing gently to adhere the crust.
5. Spray the air fryer basket with cooking spray and place the trout fillets in a single layer.
6. Cook for 8-10 minutes, depending on the thickness of the fillets, until the fish is cooked through and the crust is golden brown.
7. Serve hot with lemon wedges.

Nutritional values:

Calories: 285kcal | Fat: 18g | Protein: 28g | Carbs: 2g | Net carbs: 1g | Fiber: 1g | Cholesterol: 77mg | Sodium: 129mg | Potassium: 515mg

Air Fryer Spicy Tuna Cakes

Serving: 4 | Preparation Time: 20 minutes

Ingredients:

• 20 oz (600g) tuna, drained
• 2 oz (60g) green onions, finely chopped
• 1 oz (30 g) almond flour

- 1 tbsp Dijon mustard
- 1 tsp paprika
- 1/2 tsp garlic powder
- 1/4 tsp cayenne pepper (adjust to taste)
- Salt and pepper to taste
- Cooking spray
- Lemon wedges, for serving

Instructions:

1. In a large bowl, combine the drained tuna, chopped green onions, almond flour, Dijon mustard, paprika, garlic powder, cayenne pepper, salt, and pepper. Mix well until all the ingredients are evenly incorporated.
2. Shape the mixture into small patties, about 2-3 inches in diameter.
3. Preheat the air fryer to 375°F (190°C).
4. Spray the air fryer basket with cooking spray and place the tuna cakes in a single layer.
5. Cook for 8-10 minutes, flipping halfway through, until the cakes are golden brown and heated through.
6. Serve hot with lemon wedges on the side.

Nutritional values:
Calories: 185kcal | Fat: 6g | Protein: 26g | Carbs: 4g | Net carbs: 3g | Fiber: 1g | Cholesterol: 36mg | Sodium: 382mg | Potassium: 293mg

Air Fryer Blackened Red Snapper

Serving: 4 | Preparation Time: 15 minutes

Ingredients:

- 24 oz (720g) red snapper fillets
- 2 tbsp olive oil
- 1 tbsp paprika
- 1 tsp dried thyme
- 1 tsp dried oregano
- 1 tsp onion powder
- 1 tsp garlic powder
- 1/2 tsp cayenne pepper (adjust to taste)
- Salt and pepper to taste
- Cooking spray
- Lemon wedges, for serving

Instructions:

1. Preheat the air fryer to 375°F (190°C).
2. In a small bowl, combine paprika, dried thyme, dried oregano, onion powder, garlic powder, cayenne pepper, salt, and pepper to create the blackened seasoning.
3. Brush both sides of the red snapper fillets with olive oil.
4. Sprinkle the blackened seasoning evenly over the fillets, pressing it gently to adhere.
5. Spray the air fryer basket with cooking spray and place the seasoned red snapper fillets in a single layer.
6. Cook for 8-10 minutes, depending on the thickness of the fillets, until the fish is cooked through and the seasoning is slightly charred.
7. Serve hot with lemon wedges on the side.

Nutritional values:
Calories: 240kcal | Fat: 11g | Protein: 34g | Carbs: 2g | Net carbs: 1g | Fiber: 1g | Cholesterol: 72mg | Sodium: 165mg | Potassium: 696mg

Air Fryer Mediterranean Fish

Serving: 4 | Preparation Time: 20 minutes

Ingredients:

- 20 oz (600g) white fish fillets (such as cod or tilapia)
- 2 tbsp olive oil
- 2 cloves garlic, minced
- 1 tsp dried oregano
- 1 tsp dried basil
- 1/2 tsp paprika
- 1/4 tsp cayenne pepper (adjust to taste)
- Salt and pepper to taste
- Cooking spray
- Lemon wedges, for serving

Instructions:

1. Preheat the air fryer to 375°F (190°C).
2. In a small bowl, combine olive oil, minced garlic, dried oregano, dried basil, paprika, cayenne pepper, salt, and pepper. Stir well to make a marinade.
3. Pat dry the fish fillets using a paper towel.

4. Rub the fish fillets with the marinade, ensuring they are evenly coated.

5. Spray the air fryer basket with cooking spray to prevent sticking.

6. Place the seasoned fish fillets in a single layer in the air fryer basket.

7. Cook for 8-10 minutes, flipping halfway through, until the fish is cooked through and golden brown.

8. Once cooked, remove the fish from the air fryer.

9. Serve hot with lemon wedges on the side.

Nutritional values:

Calories: 185kcal | Fat: 6g | Protein: 26g | Carbs: 4g | Net carbs: 3g | Fiber: 1g | Cholesterol: 36mg | Sodium: 382mg | Potassium: 293mg

Air Fryer Salmon Patties

Serving: 4 | Preparation Time: 20 minutes

Ingredients:

• 15 oz (450g) salmon fillet, cooked and flaked
• 1 oz (30g) low-carb bread crumbs
• 2 oz (60g) green onions, finely chopped
• 1 oz (30g) low fat Greek yougurt
• 1 tbsp Dijon mustard
• 1 tbsp lemon juice
• 1 tsp Old Bay seasoning
• 1/2 tsp garlic powder
• 1/4 tsp salt
• 1/4 tsp black pepper
• Cooking spray
• Lemon wedges, for serving

Instructions:

1. In a large bowl, combine the cooked and flaked salmon, bread crumbs, green onions, low fat Greek yougurt, Dijon mustard, lemon juice, Old Bay seasoning, garlic powder, salt, and black pepper. Mix well until all the ingredients are evenly incorporated.

2. Shape the mixture into small patties, about 2-3 inches in diameter.

3. Preheat the air fryer to 375°F (190°C).

4. Spray the air fryer basket with cooking spray and place the salmon patties in a single layer.

5. Cook for 8-10 minutes, flipping halfway through, until the patties are golden brown and heated through.

6. Once cooked, remove the salmon patties from the air fryer.

7. Serve hot with lemon wedges on the side.

Nutritional values:

Calories: 230kcal | Fat: 14g | Protein: 19g | Carbs: 7g | Fiber: 1g | Cholesterol: 50mg | Sodium: 420mg | Potassium: 430mg

Air Fryer Fish Curry

Serving: 4 | Preparation Time: 10 minutes | Cooking Time: 15 minutes

Ingredients:

• 15 oz (450g) white fish fillets cut into bite-sized pieces
• 2 tbsp curry powder
• 1 tsp ground cumin
• 1 tsp grated fresh ginger
• 2 cloves garlic, minced
• 2 oz (60g) onion finely chopped
• 14 oz (400ml) coconut milk
• 2 tbsp vegetable oil
• Salt and pepper to taste

Instructions:

1. Preheat the air fryer to 375°F (190°C).

2. In a bowl, combine the curry powder, ground cumin, grated ginger, minced garlic, salt, and pepper.

3. Place the fish pieces in a separate bowl and sprinkle the spice mixture over them. Toss gently to coat the fish evenly with the spices.

4. Lightly brush the air fryer basket with vegetable oil to prevent sticking.

5. Arrange the fish pieces in a single layer in the air fryer basket.

6. Cook in the air fryer at 375°F (190°C) for 12-15 minutes, or until the fish is cooked through and lightly browned.

7. While the fish is cooking, heat vegetable oil in a saucepan over medium heat. Add the chopped onion and sauté until translucent.

8. Add the minced garlic and grated ginger to the saucepan and cook for another minute until fragrant.

9. Stir in the curry powder and ground cumin, cooking for an additional minute to release the flavors.

10. Pour in the coconut milk and bring the mixture to a simmer. Cook for 5 minutes, stirring occasionally.

11. Once the fish is done, transfer the cooked fish to the saucepan with the coconut milk mixture. Gently stir to combine and simmer for 2-3 minutes to allow the flavors to meld together.

12. Remove from heat and serve the Air Fryer Fish Curry hot with steamed rice or naan bread.

Nutritional values:

Calories: 300kcal | Fat: 18g | Protein: 22g | Carbohydrates: 12g | Fiber: 3g | Cholesterol: 50mg | Sodium: 230mg | Potassium: 710mg

Seafood Recipes

Air Fryer Bang Shrimp

Serving: 4 | Preparation time: 15 minutes | Cooking time: 8-10 minutes

Ingredients:

- 2.4 oz (70g) medium shrimp, peeled and deveined
- 2.4 oz (70g) wholewheat flour
- 2 oz (60ml) unsweetened almond milk
- 2 oz (60ml) low fat Greek yougurt
- 1/2 tsp garlic powder
- 2 tbsp unsalted butter, melted
- 1 tsp honey
- Salt and black pepper to taste
- Optional garnish: chopped green onions, sesame seeds

Instructions:

1. Preheat the air fryer to 375°F (190°C).
2. In a mixing bowl, toss the shrimp with whole-wheat flour until fully coated.
3. In another mixing bowl, whisk together almond milk, low fat Greek yougurt, melted butter, honey, garlic powder, salt, and black pepper until well combined.
4. Dip the coated shrimp into the sauce mixture and toss to coat.
5. Place the shrimp onto the air fryer basket, leaving space between each shrimp.
6. Air fry for 8-10 minutes, flipping the shrimp halfway through the cooking time, until the shrimp are cooked through and crispy.
7. Garnish with chopped green onions and sesame seeds, if desired.

Note: The use of too much sugar or honey might affect your sugar level, be careful of excess sugar or honey.

Nutritional values:

Calories: 392 kcal | Fat: 19g | Protein: 22g | Carbs: 33g | Net carbs: 28g | Fiber: 5g | Cholesterol: 246mg | Sodium: 1283mg | Potassium: 278mg

Air Fryer Crab Cakes

Serving: 4 | Preparation time: 15 minutes | Cooking time: 8-10 minutes

Ingredients:

- 15 oz (450g) lump crab meat, drained
- 2 oz (60g) low fat Greek yougurt
- 0.88 oz (20g) almond flour
- 0.88 oz (20g) finely chopped celery
- 0.88 oz (20g) finely chopped green onion
- 1 large egg, beaten
- 1 tbsp Dijon mustard
- 1 tbsp Worcestershire sauce (make sure it's sugar-free)
- 1 tbsp lemon juice
- Salt and black pepper, to taste
- 1/4 tsp Garlic powder
- 1/4 tsp paprika
- Lemon wedges, for serving
- 1 oz (30g) chopped parsley

Instructions:

1. Preheat the air fryer to 400°F (205°C).
2. In a mixing bowl, combine crab meat, low fat Greek yougurt, almond flour, celery, green onion, egg, Dijon mustard, Worcestershire sauce, lemon juice, garlic powder, paprika, salt, and black pepper.
3. Mix all the ingredients until well combined.
4. Form the mixture into 8 crab cakes and place them on a baking sheet.
5. Place the crab cakes into the air fryer basket and air fry for 8-10 minutes, flipping the crab cakes halfway through the cooking time, until the crab cakes are golden brown and cooked through.
6. Serve with lemon wedges and chopped parsley, if desired.

Nutritional values:

Calories: 159 kcal | Fat: 9g | Protein: 17g | Carbs: 3g | Net carbs: 2g | Fiber: 1g | Cholesterol: 98mg | Sodium: 562mg | Potassium: 242mg

Air Fryer Scallops Wrapped in Bacon

Serving: 4 | Preparation time: 10 minutes | Cooking time: 8-10 minutes

Ingredients:

• 8 oz (240g) large sea scallops
• 4 oz (120g) slices of bacon, cut in half
• 1 tbsp olive oil
• 1/2 tsp garlic powder
• 1/2 tsp paprika
• Salt and black pepper, to taste
• Optional garnish: chopped parsley

Instructions:

1. Preheat the air fryer to 375°F (190°C).
2. Rinse the scallops under cold water and pat dry with paper towels.
3. Season the scallops with olive oil, garlic powder, paprika, salt, and black pepper.
4. Wrap each scallop with a half slice of bacon, securing with a toothpick.
5. Place the scallops onto the air fryer basket, leaving space between each scallop.
6. Air fry for 8-10 minutes, flipping the scallops halfway through the cooking time, until the bacon is crispy and the scallops are cooked through.
7. Garnish with chopped parsley, if desired.

Nutritional values:

Calories: 175 kcal | Fat: 10g | Protein: 16g | Carbs: 2g | Net carbs: 2g | Fiber: 0g | Cholesterol: 39mg | Sodium: 468mg | Potassium: 321mg

Air Fryer Garlic Butter Scallops

Serving: 4 | Preparation time: 10 minutes | Cooking time: 6-8 minutes

Ingredients:

• 15 oz (450g) fresh sea scallops, rinsed and patted dry
• 2 tbsp unsalted butter, melted
• 2 cloves garlic, minced
• Salt and black pepper, to taste
• 1 tbsp fresh lemon juice
• 1 tbsp grated Parmesan cheese
• Optional garnish: chopped fresh parsley

Instructions:

1. Preheat the air fryer to 400°F (200°C).
2. In a mixing bowl, toss the scallops with melted butter, minced garlic, salt, and black pepper until well coated.
3. Place the scallops onto the air fryer basket, leaving space between each scallop.
4. Air fry for 6-8 minutes, flipping the scallops halfway through the cooking time, until the scallops are cooked through and golden brown.
5. Drizzle the scallops with fresh lemon juice and sprinkle with grated Parmesan cheese.
6. Garnish with chopped fresh parsley, if desired.

Nutritional values:

Calories: 190 kcal | Fat: 10g | Protein: 19g | Carbs: 5g | Net carbs: 4g | Fiber: 1g | Cholesterol: 56mg | Sodium: 482mg | Potassium: 328mg

Air Fryer Coconut Shrimp

Serving 4 | Preparation time: 10 minutes | Cooking time: 8-10 minutes

Ingredients:

• 15 oz (450g) large shrimp, peeled and deveined
• 2 oz (60g) almond flour
• 1/2 tsp garlic powder
• 1/2 tsp paprika
• 1/2 tsp salt
• 2 large eggs, beaten
• 2.6 oz (80g) unsweetened shredded coconut
• Cooking spray

Instructions:

1. Preheat the air fryer to 375°F (190°C).
2. In a mixing bowl, whisk together flour, garlic powder, paprika, and salt.
3. In another mixing bowl, beat the eggs.
4. Place the shredded coconut in a separate mixing bowl.
5. Dredge each shrimp in the flour mixture, then dip it into the beaten eggs, and finally coat it in shredded coconut.
6. Place the coated shrimp onto the air fryer basket, leaving space between each shrimp.
7. Spray the shrimp with cooking spray.

8. Air fry for 8-10 minutes, flipping the shrimp halfway through the cooking time, until the shrimp are cooked through and golden brown.

Nutritional values:

Calories: 310 kcal | Fat: 17g | Protein: 20g | Carbs: 20g | Net carbs: 16g | Fiber: 4g | Cholesterol: 244mg | Sodium: 764mg | Potassium: 273mg

Air Fryer Shrimp Fajitas

Serving 4 | Preparation time: 10 minutes | Cooking time: 8-10 minutes

Ingredients:

- 15 oz (450g) raw shrimp, peeled and deveined
- 2 oz (60g) red bell pepper, sliced
- 2 oz (60g) green bell pepper, sliced
- 2 oz (60g) yellow onion, sliced
- 1 tbsp olive oil
- 2 tsp chili powder
- 1 tsp ground cumin
- 1/2 tsp smoked paprika
- 1/2 tsp garlic powder
- Salt and black pepper, to taste

Instructions:

1. Preheat the air fryer to 400°F (200°C).
2. In a mixing bowl, toss the shrimp, bell peppers, and onion with olive oil, chili powder, cumin, smoked paprika, garlic powder, salt, and black pepper until well coated.
3. Place the shrimp and vegetables onto the air fryer basket, spreading them out in a single layer.
4. Air fry for 8-10 minutes, shaking the basket halfway through the cooking time, until the shrimp are pink and cooked through and the vegetables are tender and slightly charred.
5. Serve with optional toppings, such as sour cream, shredded cheese, diced tomatoes, chopped cilantro, lime wedges, tortillas, or lettuce wraps.

Nutritional values:

Calories: 194 kcal | Fat: 5g | Protein: 28g | Carbs: 9g | Net carbs: 7g | Fiber: 2g | Cholesterol: 233mg | Sodium: 439mg | Potassium: 366mg

Air Fryer Cajun Shrimp and Sausage

Serving 4 | Preparation time: 10 minutes | Cooking time: 8-10 minutes

Ingredients:

- 15 oz (450g) raw shrimp, peeled and deveined
- 15 oz (450g) smoked sausage, sliced
- 2 oz (60g) red bell pepper, sliced
- 2 oz (60g) green bell pepper, sliced
- 2 oz (60g) yellow onion, sliced
- 2 tbsp olive oil
- 1 tbsp Cajun seasoning
- Salt and pepper, to taste

Instructions:

1. Preheat the air fryer to 400°F (200°C).
2. In a large bowl, combine the shrimp, sausage, bell peppers, onion, olive oil, Cajun seasoning, salt, and pepper. Toss until well coated.
3. Transfer the mixture to the air fryer basket and spread it out in a single layer.
4. Cook for 10-12 minutes, shaking the basket halfway through, until the shrimp are pink and cooked through and the vegetables are tender and slightly charred.
5. Serve hot.

Nutritional values:

Calories: 426kcal | Fat: 32g | Protein: 23g | Carbs: 11g | Net carbs: 9g | Fiber: 2g | Cholesterol: 181mg | Sodium: 1143mg | Potassium: 388mg

Air Fryer Seafood Stuffed Mushrooms

Serving: 4 | Preparation time: 20 minutes | Cooking time: 8-10 minutes

Ingredients:

- 8 oz (240g) large mushrooms, stems removed
- 2 oz (60g) cooked shrimp, chopped
- 2 oz (60g) cooked crab meat, chopped
- 2 oz (60g) almond flour
- 1 oz (25g) grated Parmesan cheese
- 1 tbsp olive oil
- 1 tsp garlic powder
- Salt and pepper, to taste

Instructions:

1. Preheat the air fryer to 375°F (190°C).
2. In a medium mixing bowl, combine the chopped shrimp, crab meat, almond flour, grated Parmesan cheese, olive oil, garlic powder, salt, and pepper.
3. Stuff the mushroom caps with the seafood mixture.
4. Place the stuffed mushrooms in the air fryer basket and cook for 8-10 minutes or until the mushrooms are tender and the stuffing is golden brown.
5. Serve the stuffed mushrooms hot.

Nutritional values:

Calories: 104 kcal | Fat: 6g | Protein: 8g | Carbs: 5g | Net carbs: 3g | Fiber: 2g | Cholesterol: 36mg | Sodium: 238mg | Potassium: 265mg

Air Fryer Shrimp Stir Fry

Serving: 4 | Preparation time: 20 minutes | Cooking time: 10-12 minutes

Ingredients:

• 15 oz (450g) medium-sized shrimp, peeled and deveined
• 5 oz (150g) bell peppers, sliced
• 2 oz (60g) onion, sliced
• 1 tbsp olive oil
• 2 tbsp low-sodium soy sauce
• 2 tsp honey
• 1 tsp minced garlic
• 1/2 tsp ground ginger

Instructions:

1. Preheat the air fryer to 380°F (193°C).
2. In a small mixing bowl, whisk together the soy sauce, honey, minced garlic, and ground ginger.
3. In a large mixing bowl, add the shrimp, sliced bell peppers, and sliced onions.
4. Pour the soy sauce mixture over the shrimp and vegetables and toss to coat evenly.
5. Drizzle the olive oil over the mixture and toss again.
6. Place the mixture into the air fryer basket and cook for 10-12 minutes, shaking the basket halfway through.
7. Serve hot with rice or noodles.

Note: The use of too much sugar or honey might affect your sugar level, be careful of excess sugar or honey.

Nutritional values:

Calories: 275 kcal | Fat: 5g | Protein: 35g | Carbs: 22g | Net carbs: 21g | Fiber: 1g | Cholesterol: 285mg | Sodium: 887mg | Potassium: 505mg

Air Fryer Cajun Crab Legs

Serving: 4 | Preparation time: 5 minutes | Cooking time: 8-10 minutes

Ingredients:

• 15 oz (450g) crab legs
• 2 tbsp unsalted butter, melted
• 1 tbsp olive oil
• 1 tbsp Cajun seasoning
• 1/4 tsp garlic powder
• Salt and black pepper, to taste
• Lemon wedges, for serving

Instructions:

1. Preheat the air fryer to 400°F (200°C).
2. In a small mixing bowl, combine the melted butter, olive oil, Cajun seasoning, garlic powder, salt, and black pepper. Mix well.
3. Brush the crab legs with the mixture on both sides.
4. Place the crab legs in the air fryer basket, making sure they don't overlap.
5. Cook for 8-10 minutes or until heated through.
6. Serve hot with lemon wedges.

Nutritional values:

Calories: 297 kcal | Fat: 19g | Protein: 27g | Carbs: 1g | Net carbs: 1g | Fiber: 0g | Cholesterol: 134mg | Sodium: 1268mg | Potassium: 326mg

Air Fryer Garlic Butter Shrimp and Asparagus

Serving: 4 | Preparation time: 15 minutes | Cooking time: 10-12 minutes

Ingredients:

• 15 oz (450g) large raw shrimp, peeled and deveined
• 1/4 tsp salt

- 15 oz (450g) asparagus spears, trimmed
- 2 cloves garlic, minced
- 2 oz (56g) unsalted butter, melted
- 1 tbsp lemon juice
- 1/4 tsp black pepper
- 1 tbsp chopped fresh parsley

Instructions:

1. Preheat the air fryer to 400°F (200°C).
2. In a small mixing bowl, combine the minced garlic, melted butter, salt, black pepper, and lemon juice. Mix well.
3. Place the asparagus spears in the air fryer basket and brush them with the garlic butter mixture.
4. Cook for 6-8 minutes or until the asparagus is tender-crisp.
5. Remove the basket from the air fryer and add the shrimp, then brush them with the garlic butter mixture.
6. Return the basket to the air fryer and cook for an additional 3-4 minutes or until the shrimp is pink and cooked through.
7. Sprinkle with chopped parsley before serving.

Nutritional values:

Calories: 279 kcal | Fat: 18g | Protein: 22g | Carbs: 7g | Net carbs: 4g | Fiber: 3g | Cholesterol: 223mg | Sodium: 528mg | Potassium: 593mg

Air Fryer Grilled Shrimp Skewers

Serving: 4 | Preparation time: 15 minutes | Cooking time: 5-6 minutes

Ingredients:

- 15 oz (450g) large shrimp, peeled and deveined
- 2 cloves garlic, minced
- 2 tbsp olive oil
- 1 tsp smoked paprika
- 1 tsp ground cumin
- 1/2 tsp salt
- 1/4 tsp black pepper
- 1 lemon, cut into wedges
- Skewers

Instructions:

1. Preheat the air fryer to 400°F (200°C).

2. In a large mixing bowl, combine the minced garlic, olive oil, smoked paprika, ground cumin, salt and black pepper.
3. Add the shrimp to the bowl and toss to coat well with the marinade.
4. Thread the shrimp onto skewers, alternating with lemon wedges.
5. Place the skewers in the air fryer basket, making sure they don't touch each other.
6. Cook for 5-6 minutes or until the shrimp are pink and opaque.
7. Flip the skewers halfway through the cooking time.
8. Serve hot with additional lemon wedges.

Nutritional values:

Calories: 175 kcal | Fat: 10g | Protein: 20g | Carbs: 3g | Net carbs: 3g | Fiber: 0g | Cholesterol: 190mg | Sodium: 687mg | Potassium: 192mg

Air Fryer Seafood Paella

Serving: 4 | Preparation time: 20 minutes | Cooking time: 25-30 minutes

Ingredients:

- 15 oz (450g) large shrimp, peeled and deveined
- 15 oz (450g) mussels, cleaned and debearded
- 7 oz (225g) chorizo sausage, sliced
- 2 oz (60g) onion, diced
- 2 oz (60g) red bell pepper, diced
- 3 cloves garlic, minced
- 1 tsp smoked paprika
- 10 oz (300g) Arborio rice
- Salt and pepper to taste
- 1 lemon, cut into wedges

Instructions:

1. Preheat the air fryer to 375°F (190°C).
2. In a large mixing bowl, combine the sliced chorizo, diced onion, diced red bell pepper, minced garlic, smoked paprika, and arborio rice. Mix well until all ingredients are well combined.
3. Pour the mixture into the air fryer basket and spread it out evenly.
4. Cook for 5 minutes, stirring occasionally.
5. Pour the mixture into the air fryer basket and stir well.

6. Cook for another 10-12 minutes or until the rice is cooked through and the liquid is absorbed.

7. Add the shrimp and mussels to the air fryer basket. Season with salt and pepper, to taste.

8. Cook for another 8-10 minutes or until the shrimp are pink and the mussels are open.

9. Serve hot with lemon wedges on the side.

Nutritional values:

Calories: 522 kcal | Fat: 20g | Protein: 37g | Carbs: 47g | Net carbs: 46g | Fiber: 1g | Cholesterol: 200mg | Sodium: 1144mg | Potassium: 671mg

Air Fryer Crab Rangoon

Serving: 4 | Preparation Time: 20 minutes

Ingredients:

• 8 wonton wrappers
• 4 oz (113g) cream cheese, softened
• 4 oz (113g) lump crab meat, drained and flaked
• 2 oz (60g) green onions, finely chopped
• 1/2 tsp Worcestershire sauce (make sure it's sugar-free)
• 1/2 tsp less sodium soy sauce
• 1/4 tsp garlic powder
• Vegetable oil or cooking spray for greasing
• Salt and pepper to taste

Instructions:

1. In a mixing bowl, combine the softened cream cheese, crab meat, chopped green onions, Worcestershire sauce, soy sauce, salt, pepper and garlic powder. Mix well until all the ingredients are evenly incorporated.

2. Lay out the wonton wrappers on a clean surface. Place a spoonful of the cream cheese and crab mixture in the center of each wrapper.

3. Moisten the edges of the wrappers with water to help seal them. Fold the wrapper in half diagonally, forming a triangle. Press the edges firmly to seal.

4. Preheat the air fryer to 375°F (190°C).

5. Lightly grease the air fryer basket with vegetable oil or cooking spray to prevent sticking.

6. Place the stuffed crab rangoon in a single layer in the air fryer basket, making sure they are not touching each other.

7. Cook the crab rangoon in the air fryer for 6-8 minutes, or until they turn golden brown and crispy.

8. Carefully remove the crab rangoon from the air fryer and let them cool for a few minutes before serving.

9. Serve the crab rangoon with your favorite dipping sauce, such as sweet and sour sauce or soy sauce.

Note: The addition of green onions, Worcestershire sauce, soy sauce, and garlic powder enhances the flavors and provides a hint of umami. Air frying gives the crab rangoon a crispy texture without the need for deep frying.

Nutritional values:

Calories: 75kcal | Fat: 4g | Protein: 4g | Carbs: 5g | Fiber: 0g | Sugar: 0g | Sodium: 180mg | Potassium: 55mg |

Air Fryer Lobster Bisque

Serving: 4 | Preparation Time: 20 minutes | Cooking Time: 30 minutes

Ingredients:

• 6 oz (170g) lobster tails shells removed and meat chopped
• 2 tbsp unsalted butter
• 2 oz (60g) small onion, diced
• 2 cloves garlic, minced
• 2 tbsp almond flour
• 4 oz (120ml) seafood or vegetable broth
• 4 oz (120ml) heavy cream
• 1 oz (30g) tomato paste
• 1 oz (30g) dry sherry (optional)
• 1/2 tsp paprika
• 1/4 tsp dried thyme
• Salt and pepper to taste
• Chopped fresh parsley, for garnish

Instructions:

1. Preheat the air fryer to 350°F (175°C).

2. In a large skillet, melt the butter over medium heat. Add the diced onion and minced garlic and sauté until softened, about 5 minutes.

3. Add the chopped lobster meat to the skillet and cook for an additional 2 minutes, stirring occasionally.

4. Sprinkle the flour over the lobster mixture and stir well to coat.

5. Gradually pour in the seafood or vegetable broth, stirring constantly to avoid any lumps.

6. Stir in the heavy cream, tomato paste, dry sherry (if using), paprika, dried thyme, salt, and pepper.

7. Cook the mixture for about 5 minutes, until it thickens slightly.

8. Transfer the lobster mixture to an oven-safe dish that fits inside the air fryer basket.

9. Place the dish in the air fryer basket and cook at 350°F (175°C) for 25-30 minutes, or until the bisque is hot and bubbly.

10. Remove the dish from the air fryer and let it cool slightly.

11. Garnish with chopped fresh parsley before serving.

12. Ladle the lobster bisque into bowls and serve hot as a delicious appetizer or main dish.

Nutritional values:

Calories: 410kcal | Fat: 28g | Protein: 16g | Carbohydrates: 21g | Fiber: 3g | Cholesterol: 150mg | Sodium: 990mg | Potassium: 600mg

Chapter 8.
Vegetarian Recipes

Air Fryer Tofu

Serving: 4 | Preparation time: 10 minutes | Cooking time: 12-15 minutes

Ingredients:

- 14 oz (400g) extra-firm tofu
- 1 tbsp less sodium soy sauce
- 1 tbsp olive oil
- 1 tsp garlic powder
- 1 tsp paprika
- Salt and black pepper, to taste

Instructions:

1. Preheat the air fryer to 375°F (190°C).
2. Drain the tofu and pat it dry with paper towels.
3. Cut the tofu into 1-inch (2.5cm) cubes.
4. In a mixing bowl, whisk together the soy sauce, olive oil, garlic powder, and paprika.
5. Add the tofu cubes to the bowl and toss to coat them evenly with the mixture.
6. Season with salt and black pepper.
7. Place the tofu cubes in the air fryer basket in a single layer, leaving some space between them.
8. Cook for 12-15 minutes or until the tofu is crispy on the outside and tender on the inside.
9. Flip the tofu cubes halfway through the cooking time.
10. Remove from the air fryer and let them cool for a minute before serving.

Nutritional values:

Calories: 136 kcal | Fat: 9g | Protein: 11g | Carbs: 2g | Net carbs: 1g | Fiber: 1g | Cholesterol: 0mg | Sodium: 372mg | Potassium: 84mg

Air Fryer Stuffed Peppers

Serving: 4 | Preparation time: 15 minutes | Cooking time: 20 minutes

Ingredients:

- 10 oz (300g) bell peppers
- 1 onion
- 1 garlic clove
- 1 tsp Italian seasoning
- 4 oz (120g) tomato sauce
- 1.88 oz (50g) shredded cheddar cheese
- Salt and Pepper to taste

Instructions:

1. Preheat the air fryer to 375°F (190°C).
2. Cut off the tops of the bell peppers and remove the seeds and membranes.
3. In a large skillet, add the chopped onion, minced garlic, Italian seasoning, salt and pepper and tomato sauce and cook for an additional 5-7 minutes until the vegetables are tender.
4. Stuff the bell peppers with the vegetable mixture.
5. Sprinkle the shredded cheese on top of the stuffed peppers.
6. Place the stuffed peppers in the air fryer basket.
7. Cook for 15-20 minutes or until the peppers are tender and the cheese is melted.
8. Remove from the air fryer and let them cool for a minute before serving.

Vegan Option:

Vegan cheese or omitting cheese altogether.

Nutritional values:

Calories: 322 kcal | Fat: 19g | Protein: 24g | Carbs: 15g | Net carbs: 9g | Fiber: 6g | Cholesterol: 81mg | Sodium: 559mg | Potassium: 926mg

Air Fryer Sweet Potato Fries

Serving: 4 | Preparation time: 10 minutes | Cooking time: 15-18 minutes

Ingredients:

- 7 oz (210g) sweet potatoes
- 1 tbsp olive oil
- 1 tsp garlic powder
- 1 tsp paprika
- Salt and pepper to taste

Instructions:

1. Preheat the air fryer to 400°F (200°C).
2. Wash and peel the sweet potatoes. Cut them into thin fries or wedges.
3. In a bowl, toss the sweet potato fries with olive oil, garlic powder, paprika, salt, and pepper until evenly coated.
4. Place the seasoned sweet potato fries in the air fryer basket in a single layer.
5. Cook for 15-18 minutes, shaking the basket every 5 minutes, until the sweet potato fries are crispy and golden brown.
6. Remove the sweet potato fries from the air fryer and serve immediately.

Nutritional values:
Calories: 142 kcal | Fat: 4g | Protein: 2g | Carbs: 25g | Net carbs: 21g | Fiber: 4g | Cholesterol: 0mg | Sodium: 74mg | Potassium: 438mg

Air Fryer Veggie Burger

Serving: 4 | Preparation time: 5 minutes | Cooking time: 8-10 minutes

Ingredients:

• 15 oz (453g) veggie burger patties
• 8 oz (240g) whole wheat burger buns
• 6 oz (170g) tomato, sliced
• 2 oz (60g) lettuce leaves
• 8 oz (240g) avocado, sliced
• Salt and pepper to taste
• Ketchup, mustard (optional)

Instructions:

1. Preheat the air fryer to 400°F (200°C).
2. Place the veggie burger patties in the air fryer basket.
3. Cook for 8-10 minutes, flipping halfway through, until the patties are heated through and crispy on the outside.
4. Assemble the burgers by placing a veggie burger patty on the bottom half of each burger bun, followed by a slice of tomato, a lettuce leaf, and a few slices of avocado. Season with salt and pepper to taste.
5. Add ketchup, mustard to the top half of each burger bun (optional).
6. Serve the veggie burgers immediately.

Vegan option:
Use vegan-friendly burger buns and veggie burger patties.

Nutritional values:
Calories: 293 kcal | Fat: 11g | Protein: 12g | Carbs: 37g | Net carbs: 25g | Fiber: 12g | Cholesterol: 0mg | Sodium: 527mg | Potassium: 800mg

Air Fryer Stuffed Portobello Mushrooms

Serving: 4 | Preparation time: 10 minutes | Cooking time: 10-12 minutes

Ingredients:

• 4 large portobello mushroom caps
• 1.8 oz (50g) chopped spinach
• 2.5 oz (75g) diced tomatoes
• 1.8 oz (50g) diced onion
• 1.8 oz (50g) diced bell pepper
• 1.8 oz (50g) crumbled feta cheese
• 2 cloves garlic, minced
• Salt and pepper to taste
• 1 tbsp olive oil
• Chopped fresh parsley for garnish

Instructions:

1. Preheat the air fryer to 375°F (190°C).
2. Remove the stems and gills from the mushroom caps and brush the caps with olive oil.
3. In a bowl, mix together the spinach, tomatoes, onion, bell pepper, feta cheese, garlic, salt, and pepper.
4. Divide the mixture evenly between the mushroom caps, pressing down gently to fill them.
5. Place the stuffed mushroom caps in the air fryer basket.
6. Cook for 10-12 minutes, or until the mushrooms are tender and the filling is heated through.
7. Garnish with chopped fresh parsley and serve immediately.

Vegan option:
Use vegan-friendly cheese or omit the cheese altogether.

Nutritional values:
Calories: 100 kcal | Fat: 5g | Protein: 5g | Carbs: 11g | Net carbs: 8g | Fiber: 3g | Cholesterol: 11mg | Sodium: 210mg | Potassium: 580mg

Air Fryer Cauliflower Steaks

Serving: 4 | Preparation time: 10 minutes | Cooking time: 10-12 minutes

Ingredients:
• 20 oz (600g) cauliflower
• 1 tbsp olive oil
• 1 tsp smoked paprika
• 1/2 tsp garlic powder
• Salt and black pepper, to taste

Instructions:
1. Preheat the air fryer to 375°F (190°C).
2. Remove the leaves from the cauliflower and trim the stem.
3. Slice the cauliflower into 1-inch (2.5cm) thick steaks.
4. In a small bowl, mix together the olive oil, smoked paprika, garlic powder, salt, and black pepper.
5. Brush both sides of the cauliflower steaks with the spice mixture.
6. Place the cauliflower steaks in the air fryer basket in a single layer, leaving some space between them.
7. Cook for 10-12 minutes or until the cauliflower is tender and slightly charred on the outside.
8. Flip the cauliflower steaks halfway through the cooking time.
9. Remove from the air fryer and serve hot.

Vegan Option:
By using vegan butter or olive oil this recipe becomes suitable for a vegan diet.

Nutritional values:
Calories: 66 kcal | Fat: 4g | Protein: 2g | Carbs: 7g | Net carbs: 4g | Fiber: 3g | Cholesterol: 0mg | Sodium: 52mg | Potassium: 430mg

Air Fryer Roasted Brussel Sprouts

Serving: 4 | Preparation time: 5 minutes | Cooking time: 10-12 minutes

Ingredients:
• 15 oz (450g) brussel sprouts, trimmed and halved
• 2 tbsp olive oil
• 1 tsp garlic powder
• Salt and black pepper, to taste

Instructions:
1. Preheat the air fryer to 400°F (200°C).
2. In a bowl, mix together the brussel sprouts, olive oil, garlic powder, salt, and black pepper.
3. Toss until the brussel sprouts are coated evenly.
4. Place the brussel sprouts in the air fryer basket in a single layer, leaving some space between them.
5. Cook for 10-12 minutes or until the brussel sprouts are tender and slightly browned on the outside.
6. Shake the basket every 4 minutes to ensure even cooking.
7. Remove from the air fryer and serve hot.

Nutritional values:
Calories: 118 kcal | Fat: 8g | Protein: 3g | Carbs: 11g | Net carbs: 7g | Fiber: 4g | Cholesterol: 0mg | Sodium: 46mg | Potassium: 494mg

Air Fryer Asparagus

Serving: 4 | Preparation time: 5 minutes | Cooking time: 8-10 minutes

Ingredients:
• 15 oz (450g) asparagus, woody ends trimmed
• 1 tbsp olive oil
• Salt and black pepper, to taste
• 1/2 tsp garlic powder
• 1/4 tsp onion powder

Instructions:
1. Preheat the air fryer to 375°F (190°C).
2. In a mixing bowl, toss the asparagus with olive oil, salt, black pepper, garlic powder, and onion powder until evenly coated.

3. Place the asparagus in the air fryer basket in a single layer.

4. Cook for 8-10 minutes or until the asparagus is tender and slightly charred on the outside.

5. Shake the basket halfway through the cooking time to ensure even cooking.

6. Remove the asparagus from the air fryer and serve hot.

Nutritional values:

Calories: 57 kcal | Fat: 4g | Protein: 2g | Carbs: 5g | Net carbs: 3g | Fiber: 2g | Cholesterol: 0mg | Sodium: 85mg | Potassium: 239mg

Air Fryer Zucchini Fries

Serving: 4 | Preparation time: 15 minutes | Cooking time: 10-12 minutes

Ingredients:

- 7 oz (210g) zucchinis
- 1 oz (30g) almond flour
- 0.88 oz (25g) grated parmesan cheese
- 1/2 tsp garlic powder
- 1/2 tsp onion powder
- 1/4 tsp salt
- 1/4 tsp black pepper
- 1 large egg, beaten
- Cooking spray

Instructions:

1. Preheat the air fryer to 400°F (200°C).

2. Cut the zucchinis into thin sticks, about 1/2-inch (1.25cm) thick and 3-4 inches (7-10cm) long.

3. In a shallow dish, mix together the almond flour, grated parmesan cheese, garlic powder, onion powder, salt, and black pepper.

4. In another shallow dish, beat the egg.

5. Dip each zucchini stick into the beaten egg, then into the almond flour mixture, making sure it is well coated.

6. Place the zucchini sticks in the air fryer basket in a single layer, leaving some space between them.

7. Spray the zucchini sticks with cooking spray.

8. Cook for 10-12 minutes or until golden brown and crispy.

9. Flip the zucchini sticks halfway through the cooking time.

10. Remove from the air fryer and serve hot with your favorite dipping sauce.

Vegan option:

Substitute the egg with a flax or chia egg. To make a flax or chia egg, mix 1 tbsp of ground flax or chia seeds with 3 tbsp of water and let it sit for 5-10 minutes until it forms a gel.

Nutritional values:

Calories: 140 kcal | Fat: 9g | Protein: 8g | Carbs: 8g | Net carbs: 4g | Fiber: 4g | Cholesterol: 63mg | Sodium: 322mg | Potassium: 418mg

Air Fryer Roasted Carrots

Serving: 4 | Preparation time: 10 minutes | Cooking time: 10-12 minutes

Ingredients:

- 15 oz (450g) carrots, peeled and cut into 1/2-inch (1.25cm) thick rounds
- 1 tbsp olive oil
- 1/2 tsp garlic powder
- 1/2 tsp onion powder
- 1/2 tsp dried thyme
- 1/4 tsp salt
- 1/4 tsp black pepper

Instructions:

1. Preheat the air fryer to 400°F (200°C).

2. In a large bowl, mix together the olive oil, garlic powder, onion powder, dried thyme, salt, and black pepper.

3. Add the carrot rounds to the bowl and toss until the carrots are well coated with the seasoning mixture.

4. Place the seasoned carrots in the air fryer basket in a single layer, leaving some space between them.

5. Cook for 10-12 minutes or until the carrots are tender and lightly browned, flipping them halfway through the cooking time.

6. Remove from the air fryer and serve hot.

Nutritional values:
Calories: 90 kcal | Fat: 4g | Protein: 1g | Carbs: 13g | Net carbs: 9g | Fiber: 4g | Cholesterol: 0mg | Sodium: 236mg | Potassium: 409mg

Air Fryer Kale Chips

Serving: 4 | Preparation Time: 15 minutes

Ingredients:

• 8 oz (240g) of kale
• 1 tbsp olive oil
• Salt to taste
• Optional seasonings: garlic powder, paprika, nutritional yeast, etc.

Instructions:

1. Preheat the air fryer to 375°F (190°C).
2. Wash and thoroughly dry the kale leaves. Remove the tough stems and tear the leaves into bite-sized pieces.
3. In a large bowl, drizzle the kale with olive oil and sprinkle with salt. Toss well to coat the leaves evenly.
4. If desired, add any additional seasonings or spices of your choice, such as garlic powder, paprika, or nutritional yeast. Toss again to distribute the seasonings.
5. Place the seasoned kale leaves in the air fryer basket in a single layer. You may need to cook them in batches depending on the size of your air fryer.
6. Cook for 5-7 minutes, shaking the basket halfway through, until the kale chips are crispy and lightly browned. Keep a close eye on them to prevent burning.
7. Remove the kale chips from the air fryer and let them cool for a few minutes before serving. They will become even crispier as they cool.

Note: Feel free to experiment with different seasonings to customize the flavor of your kale chips. Enjoy them as a healthy and crunchy snack!

Nutritional values:
Calories: 50kcal | Fat: 3g | Protein: 2g | Carbs: 5g | Net carbs: 3g | Fiber: 2g | Sodium: 60mg | Potassium: 370mg |

Air Fryer Garlic Mushrooms

Serving: 4 | Preparation Time: 15 minutes

Ingredients:

• 15 oz (450g) button mushrooms
• 2 tbsp olive oil
• 4 cloves garlic, minced
• 1 tbsp balsamic vinegar
• Salt and pepper to taste
• Fresh parsley, chopped, for garnish

Instructions:

1. Preheat the air fryer to 375°F (190°C).
2. Clean the mushrooms and trim the stems if necessary. If the mushrooms are large, you can halve or quarter them.
3. In a bowl, combine the olive oil or melted vegan butter, minced garlic, balsamic vinegar, salt, and pepper. Mix well.
4. Add the mushrooms to the bowl and toss until they are evenly coated with the garlic mixture.
5. Place the mushrooms in the air fryer basket in a single layer. You may need to cook them in batches depending on the size of your air fryer.
6. Cook for 10-12 minutes, shaking the basket halfway through, until the mushrooms are tender and golden brown.
7. Remove from the air fryer and garnish with fresh parsley before serving.

Nutritional values:
Calories: 120kcal | Fat: 8g | Protein: 3g | Carbs: 9g | Net carbs: 6g | Fiber: 3g | Cholesterol: 0mg | Sodium: 10mg | Potassium: 700mg

Air Fryer Eggplant Parmesan

Serving: 4 | Preparation Time: 25 minutes

Ingredients:

• 1 large eggplant
• 4 oz (120g) low-carb breadcrumbs
• 2 oz (60g) grated Parmesan cheese
• 1 tsp dried oregano
• 1 tsp dried basil
• 1/2 tsp garlic powder
• 1/2 tsp salt
• 1/4 tsp black pepper

- 2 large eggs (or flax eggs for vegan option)
- 8 oz (240ml) marinara sauce
- 4 oz (120g) shredded mozzarella cheese
- Fresh basil leaves, for garnish

Instructions:

1. Preheat the air fryer to 375°F (190°C).

2. Slice the eggplant into 1/2-inch thick rounds. If desired, you can peel the skin off the eggplant before slicing.

3. In a shallow dish, combine the breadcrumbs, grated Parmesan cheese, dried oregano, dried basil, garlic powder, salt, and black pepper. Mix well.

4. In a separate bowl, beat the eggs until well combined.

5. Dip each eggplant slice into the beaten eggs, allowing any excess to drip off, and then coat it with the breadcrumb mixture. Press the breadcrumbs gently onto each slice to ensure they adhere.

6. Place the coated eggplant slices in the air fryer basket in a single layer. You may need to cook them in batches depending on the size of your air fryer.

7. Cook for 10-12 minutes, flipping the eggplant slices halfway through, until they are golden brown and crispy.

8. Remove the cooked eggplant slices from the air fryer and set aside.

9. Spoon a tablespoon of marinara sauce onto each eggplant slice and sprinkle with shredded mozzarella cheese.

10. Return the eggplant slices to the air fryer and cook for an additional 3-5 minutes, until the cheese is melted and bubbly.

11. Remove from the air fryer and garnish with fresh basil leaves before serving.

Vegan Option:

For a vegan version, use flax eggs instead of regular eggs and substitute vegan Parmesan and mozzarella cheese.

Note: Serve the air fryer eggplant Parmesan with a side of pasta or a fresh salad for a complete meal.

Nutritional values:

Calories: 250kcal | Fat: 10g | Protein: 12g | Carbs: 29g | Net carbs: 25g | Fiber: 4g | Cholesterol: 0mg | Sodium: 800mg | Potassium: 600mg

Air Fryer Stuffed Squash

Serving: 4 | Preparation Time: 30 minutes

Ingredients:

- 2 small acorn squash
- 5 oz (160g) quinoa, cooked
- 2.5 oz (75g) diced bell peppers
- 2.5 oz (70g) diced zucchini
- 2.3 oz (70g) diced onion
- 2.3 oz (70g) diced mushrooms
- 1 oz (30g) crumbled feta cheese
- 2 tbsp olive oil
- 1 tsp dried thyme
- 1 tsp garlic powder
- Salt and pepper to taste
- Fresh parsley, chopped, for garnish

Instructions:

1. Preheat the air fryer to 375°F (190°C).

2. Cut the acorn squash in half lengthwise and scoop out the seeds and pulp.

3. In a bowl, combine the cooked quinoa, diced bell peppers, diced zucchini, diced onion, diced mushrooms, crumbled feta cheese (or vegan feta), olive oil, dried thyme, garlic powder, salt, and pepper. Mix well.

4. Fill each acorn squash half with the quinoa mixture, pressing it down gently.

5. Place the stuffed squash halves in the air fryer basket, cut side up.

6. Cook for 20-25 minutes, or until the squash is tender and the filling is heated through.

7. Remove from the air fryer and garnish with fresh parsley before serving.

Vegan Option:

To make this recipe vegan, use vegan feta cheese or omit the cheese altogether.

Note: Stuffed squash makes a satisfying and nutritious meal on its own, but you can also serve it with a side salad for a complete and balanced dinner.

Nutritional values:
Calories: 280kcal | Fat: 10g | Protein: 8g | Carbs: 45g | Net carbs: 36g | Fiber: 9g | Cholesterol: 0mg | Sodium: 160mg | Potassium: 1100mg

Air Fryer Baked Apples

Serving: 4 | Preparation Time: 20 minutes

Ingredients:

- 4 medium-sized apples (such as Granny Smith or Honeycrisp)
- 2 tbsp unsalted butter
- 2 tsp honey
- 1 tsp ground cinnamon
- 1/4 tsp ground nutmeg
- 1 oz (30g) chopped nuts (such as walnuts or pecans)
- Optional toppings: Greek yogurt, whipped cream, or vanilla ice cream (use dairy-free alternatives for vegan or lactose-free options)

Instructions:

1. Preheat the air fryer to 375°F (190°C).
2. Wash and core the apples, leaving the bottoms intact.
3. In a small bowl, mix together the butter (or coconut oil), honey (or sugar substitute), cinnamon, nutmeg, and chopped nuts.
4. Stuff the hollowed-out center of each apple with the butter and sugar mixture.
5. Place the stuffed apples in the air fryer basket.
6. Cook for 12-15 minutes, or until the apples are tender and the filling is caramelized.
7. Remove from the air fryer and let them cool slightly before serving.
8. Serve the baked apples as they are or with optional toppings like Greek yogurt, whipped cream, or vanilla ice cream.

Vegan Option:
Use coconut oil instead of butter and a sugar substitute instead of brown sugar. Choose dairy-free toppings like coconut yogurt or dairy-free ice cream.

Note: The use of too much sugar or honey might affect your sugar level, be careful of excess sugar or honey.

Air Fryer Cinnamon Sweet Potato Fries

Serving: 4 | Preparation Time: 25 minutes

Ingredients:

- 2 medium-sized sweet potatoes
- 1 tbsp olive oil
- 1 tsp ground cinnamon
- 1/2 tsp salt
- Optional: 1-2 tbsp (15-30ml) maple syrup for a sweeter taste

Instructions:

1. Preheat the air fryer to 400°F (200°C).
2. Peel the sweet potatoes and cut them into evenly sized fries, about 1/4-inch thick.
3. In a bowl, toss the sweet potato fries with olive oil, ground cinnamon, and salt. Optional: Drizzle with maple syrup for added sweetness.
4. Place the seasoned sweet potato fries in the air fryer basket in a single layer, making sure they are not overcrowded.
5. Cook for 15-20 minutes, shaking the basket or flipping the fries halfway through, until they are crispy and golden brown.
6. Remove the fries from the air fryer and let them cool for a few minutes before serving.

Vegan Option:
Ensure you choose a vegan-friendly maple syrup if using.

Note: These cinnamon sweet potato fries are a delicious and healthier alternative to traditional fries. They make a great side dish or snack. Adjust the seasoning and sweetness according to your taste preferences.

Nutritional values:
Calories: 160kcal | Fat: 4g | Protein: 2g | Carbs: 30g | Fiber: 5g | Sugar: 6g | Sodium: 315mg | Potassium: 450mg

Air Fryer Ratatouille

Serving: 4 | Preparation Time: 15 minutes | Cooking Time: 25 minutes

Ingredients:

- 15 oz (450g) eggplant, diced
- 7 oz (210g) zucchini, diced
- 4 oz (120g) red bell pepper, diced
- 4 oz (120g) yellow bell pepper, diced
- 2 oz (60g) small onion, diced
- 2 cloves garlic, minced
- 2 tbsp olive oil
- Salt and pepper to taste

Instructions:

1. Preheat the air fryer to 375°F (190°C).
2. In a large bowl, combine the diced eggplant, zucchini, red bell pepper, yellow bell pepper, onion, and minced garlic.
3. Drizzle the olive oil over the vegetables and season with salt and pepper. Toss well to coat the vegetables evenly.
4. Place the seasoned vegetables in the air fryer basket in a single layer.
5. Cook in the air fryer at 375°F (190°C) for 20-25 minutes, shaking the basket or stirring the vegetables halfway through, until they are tender and lightly browned.
6. Once the vegetables are cooked, transfer them to a serving dish.
7. Serve the Air Fryer Ratatouille as a side dish or as a main course with crusty bread or cooked grains.

Nutritional values:

Calories: 120kcal | Fat: 7g | Protein: 2g | Carbohydrates: 15g | Fiber: 5g | Cholesterol: 0mg | Sodium: 10mg | Potassium: 480mg

Air Fryer Garlic Green Beans

Serving: 4 | Preparation Time: 10 minutes | Cooking Time: 10 minutes

Ingredients:

- 15 oz (450g) fresh green beans, ends trimmed
- 2 tbsp olive oil
- 4 cloves garlic, minced
- 1/2 tsp salt
- 1/4 tsp black pepper
- Optional: crushed red pepper flakes (for added spice)

Instructions:

1. Preheat the air fryer to 375°F (190°C).
2. In a mixing bowl, combine the green beans, olive oil, minced garlic, salt, black pepper, and crushed red pepper flakes (if desired). Toss well to coat the green beans evenly.
3. Place the seasoned green beans in the air fryer basket in a single layer.
4. Cook in the air fryer at 375°F (190°C) for 8-10 minutes, shaking the basket or stirring the green beans halfway through, until they are tender-crisp and slightly charred.
5. Once the green beans are cooked, transfer them to a serving dish.
6. Serve the Air Fryer Garlic Green Beans as a delicious side dish or as a healthy snack.

Note: Omit the optional crushed red pepper flakes or use a vegan-friendly alternative for added spice.

Nutritional values:

Calories: 90kcal | Fat: 7g | Protein: 1g | Carbohydrates: 7g | Fiber: 3g | Cholesterol: 0mg | Sodium: 300mg | Potassium: 239mg

Air Fryer Onion Rings

Serving: 4 | Preparation Time: 15 minutes | Cooking Time: 15 minutes

Ingredients:

- 8 oz (240g) onions
- 4 oz (120g) almond flour
- 1 tsp paprika
- 1/2 tsp garlic powder
- 1/2 tsp salt
- 1/4 tsp black pepper
- 6 oz (180ml) plant-based milk (such as almond milk or soy milk)
- 2 oz (60g) low-carb bread crumbs (regular or panko)
- Cooking spray

Instructions:

1. Preheat the air fryer to 400°F (200°C).

2. Peel the onions and cut them into 1/2-inch thick slices. Separate the slices into rings and set aside.

3. In a shallow bowl, whisk together the almond flour, paprika, garlic powder, salt, and black pepper.

4. Pour the plant-based milk into another shallow bowl.

5. Place the bread crumbs in a third shallow bowl.

6. Take an onion ring and dip it into the flour mixture, ensuring it's coated evenly. Shake off any excess flour.

7. Dip the flour-coated onion ring into the plant-based milk, allowing any excess milk to drip off.

8. Finally, coat the onion ring with bread crumbs, pressing gently to adhere the crumbs to the ring. Repeat this process for the remaining onion rings.

9. Lightly spray the air fryer basket with cooking spray.

10. Place the coated onion rings in a single layer in the air fryer basket, without overcrowding.

11. Cook in the air fryer at 400°F (200°C) for 10-15 minutes, flipping the onion rings halfway through, until they are golden brown and crispy.

12. Once cooked, remove the onion rings from the air fryer and repeat the cooking process with any remaining onion rings.

13. Serve the Air Fryer Onion Rings immediately as a tasty appetizer or as a side dish with your favorite dipping sauce.

Vegan Option:
Use plant-based milk, such as almond milk or soy milk, instead of dairy milk. Ensure the bread crumbs used are free from any animal-derived ingredients.

Nutritional values:
Calories: 160kcal | Fat: 2g | Protein: 4g | Carbohydrates: 33g | Fiber: 3g | Cholesterol: 0mg | Sodium: 460mg | Potassium: 170mg

Air Fryer Okra

Serving: 4 | Preparation Time: 15 minutes | Cooking Time: 15 minutes

Ingredients:
• 15 oz (450g) fresh okra
• 2 tbsp olive oil
• 1 tsp ground cumin
• 1/2 tsp paprika
• 1/2 tsp garlic powder
• 1/2 tsp onion powder
• 1/4 tsp cayenne pepper
• Salt and pepper to taste

Instructions:
1. Preheat your air fryer to 400°F (200°C).

2. Wash the okra thoroughly and pat dry with a paper towel. Trim the ends of the okra pods and slice them into 1/2-inch pieces.

3. In a mixing bowl, combine the sliced okra, olive oil or vegetable oil (depending on the vegan option you prefer), ground cumin, paprika, garlic powder, onion powder, cayenne pepper, salt, and pepper. Toss everything together until the okra is evenly coated with the seasonings.

4. Place the seasoned okra in the air fryer basket in a single layer. You may need to cook them in batches depending on the size of your air fryer.

5. Air fry the okra at 400°F (200°C) for 8-10 minutes, shaking the basket halfway through to ensure even cooking.

6. Once the okra turns crispy and lightly browned, remove them from the air fryer.

Nutritional values:
Calories: 120 kcal | Fat: 8g | Saturated Fat: 1g | Trans Fat: 0g | Sodium: 10mg | Carbohydrates: 10g | Fiber: 4g | Sugars: 1g | Protein: 2g

Chapter 9. Appetizers

Air Fryer Garlic and Herb Roasted Chickpeas

Serving: 4 | Preparation time: 5 minutes | Cooking time: 12-15 minutes

Ingredients:

- 15 oz (450g) chickpeas, drained and rinsed
- 1 tbsp olive oil
- 1/2 tsp garlic powder
- 1/2 tsp dried thyme
- 1/2 tsp dried rosemary
- 1/2 tsp dried oregano
- 1/2 tsp salt
- 1/4 tsp black pepper

Instructions:

1. Preheat the air fryer to 390°F (200°C).
2. Spread the chickpeas out on a paper towel and pat them dry.
3. In a mixing bowl, combine the olive oil, garlic powder, thyme, rosemary, oregano, salt, and black pepper.
4. Add the chickpeas to the bowl and toss until they are well coated in the herb mixture.
5. Place the chickpeas in the air fryer basket in a single layer.
6. Cook for 12-15 minutes or until the chickpeas are golden brown and crispy, shaking the basket every 5 minutes to ensure even cooking.
7. Remove the chickpeas from the air fryer and let them cool for a few minutes before serving.

Nutritional values:

Calories: 171 kcal | Fat: 5g | Protein: 7g | Carbs: 25g | Net carbs: 19g | Fiber: 6g | Cholesterol: 0mg | Sodium: 316mg | Potassium: 317mg

Air Fryer Avocado Fries

Serving: 4 | Preparation time: 15 minutes | Cooking time: 7-8 minutes

Ingredients:

- 7 oz (210g) ripe avocados
- 2 oz (60g) almond flour
- 1 oz (28g) coconut flour
- 1 tsp garlic powder
- 1/2 tsp paprika
- 1/2 tsp salt
- 2 large eggs, beaten
- Cooking spray

Instructions:

1. Preheat the air fryer to 400°F (200°C).
2. Cut the avocados in half, remove the pit and peel off the skin. Slice each avocado half into 4-5 wedges.
3. In a mixing bowl, whisk together the almond flour, coconut flour, garlic powder, paprika, and salt.
4. Dip each avocado wedge into the beaten eggs and then coat it in the flour mixture.
5. Place the avocado wedges in a single layer in the air fryer basket, and spray them lightly with cooking spray.
6. Cook for 7-8 minutes or until the avocado fries are crispy and golden, flipping them halfway through cooking to ensure even cooking.
7. Remove the avocado fries from the air fryer and serve immediately with your favorite dipping sauce.

Nutritional values:

Calories: 276 kcal | Fat: 24g | Protein: 8g | Carbs: 16g | Net carbs: 5g | Fiber: 11g | Cholesterol: 93mg | Sodium: 439mg | Potassium: 671mg

Air Fryer Bacon Wrapped Asparagus

Serving: 4 | Preparation time: 10 minutes | Cooking time: 10-12 minutes

Ingredients:

• 15 oz (450g) asparagus spears, trimmed

• 8 oz (240g) slices of chicken bacon

• Salt and pepper to taste

• Cooking spray

Instructions:

1. Preheat the air fryer to 375°F (190°C).

2. Wrap each asparagus spear with one slice of bacon, starting at the base and working your way to the top.

3. Place the bacon-wrapped asparagus spears in the air fryer basket in a single layer, leaving some space between them.

4. Lightly spray the asparagus spears with cooking spray and season with salt and pepper to taste.

5. Cook for 10-12 minutes or until the bacon is crispy and the asparagus is tender, flipping the asparagus halfway through cooking.

6. Once done, remove from the air fryer and serve hot.

Nutritional values:

Calories: 191 kcal | Fat: 14g | Protein: 8g | Carbs: 7g | Net carbs: 4g | Fiber: 3g | Cholesterol: 24mg | Sodium: 395mg | Potassium: 353mg

Air Fryer Spinach and Feta Stuffed Mushrooms

Serving: 4 | Preparation time: 15 minutes | Cooking time: 10-12 minutes

Ingredients:

• 15 oz (450g) large white mushrooms, stems removed and clean

• 0.88 oz (25g) chopped spinach

• 1 oz (35g) crumbled feta cheese

• 2 tbsp olive oil

• 1/4 tsp garlic powder

• Salt and pepper to taste

• Cooking spray

Instructions:

1. Preheat the air fryer to 375°F (190°C).

2. In a small bowl, mix together the chopped spinach, crumbled feta cheese, olive oil, garlic powder, salt, and pepper until well combined.

3. Stuff each mushroom cap with the spinach and feta mixture.

4. Lightly spray the stuffed mushrooms with cooking spray and place them in the air fryer basket in a single layer.

5. Cook for 10-12 minutes or until the mushrooms are tender and the filling is golden brown and crispy.

6. Once done, remove from the air fryer and serve hot.

Nutritional values:

Calories: 77 kcal | Fat: 6g | Protein: 3g | Carbs: 3g | Net carbs: 2g | Fiber: 1g | Cholesterol: 8mg | Sodium: 88mg | Potassium: 233mg

Air Fryer Mini Meatballs with Marinara Sauce

Serving: 4 | Preparation time: 20 minutes | Cooking time: 10-12 minutes

Ingredients:

• 15 oz (450g) ground beef

• 0.88 oz (25g) grated parmesan cheese

• 0.70 oz (20g) almond flour

• 1 egg

• 1/2 tsp garlic powder

• 1/2 tsp onion powder

• Salt and pepper to taste

• 8 oz (240ml) marinara sauce

• Cooking spray

Instructions:

1. In a large bowl, mix together the ground beef, grated parmesan cheese, almond flour, egg, garlic powder, onion powder, salt, and pepper until well combined.

2. Using a small cookie scoop or spoon, form the meat mixture into small, bite-sized balls.

3. Preheat the air fryer to 375°F (190°C).

4. Lightly spray the air fryer basket with cooking spray and place the meatballs in a single layer.

5. Cook for 10-12 minutes or until the meatballs are browned and cooked through, flipping halfway through.

6. Once the meatballs are done, remove them from the air fryer and place them in a small bowl.

7. In a separate microwave-safe bowl, heat the marinara sauce in the microwave for 1-2 minutes or until heated through.

8. Serve the meatballs with the warm marinara sauce for dipping.

Nutritional values:

Calories: 274 kcal | Fat: 19g | Protein: 19g | Carbs: 6g | Net carbs: 4g | Fiber: 2g | Cholesterol: 105mg | Sodium: 578mg | Potassium: 417mg

Air Fryer Mini Vegetable Spring Rolls

Serving: 4 | Preparation time: 20 minutes | Cooking time: 8-10 minutes

Ingredients:

• 5 oz (150g) mini spring roll wrappers
• 5 oz (150g) shredded cabbage
• 2.5 oz (70g) shredded carrots
• 2.5 oz (70g) sliced mushrooms
• 1 oz (35g) chopped onions
• 1 oz (30g) chopped bell peppers
• 1 tbsp less sodium soy sauce
• 1 tsp sesame oil
• 1 tsp wholewheat flour
• Salt and pepper to taste
• Cooking spray

Instructions:

1. In a mixing bowl, combine the shredded cabbage, shredded carrots, sliced mushrooms, chopped onions, chopped bell peppers, soy sauce, sesame oil, wholewheat flour, salt, and pepper. Mix well until the vegetables are coated evenly with the sauce.

2. Lay a spring roll wrapper on a clean surface with one corner facing you. Place 1-2 tablespoons of the vegetable mixture in the center of the wrapper.

3. Fold the corner closest to you over the filling, then fold in the sides and roll up tightly. Repeat with the remaining wrappers and filling.

4. Preheat the air fryer to 350°F (180°C).

5. Place the spring rolls in the air fryer basket, leaving some space between them. Lightly spray with cooking spray.

6. Cook for 8-10 minutes or until the spring rolls are crispy and golden brown, flipping them halfway through cooking.

7. Once done, remove from the air fryer and serve hot with your favorite dipping sauce.

Nutritional values:

Calories: 50 kcal | Fat: 0.9g | Protein: 1.3g | Carbs: 9.2g | Net carbs: 8.2g | Fiber: 1g | Cholesterol: 0mg | Sodium: 200mg | Potassium: 87mg

Air Fryer Stuffed Peppers with Ground Turkey

Serving: 4 | Preparation time: 15 minutes | Cooking time: 18-20 minutes

Ingredients:

• 4 oz (120g) large bell peppers
• 15 oz (450g) lean ground turkey
• 4 oz (120g) cooked rice (white)
• 2 oz (60g) diced tomatoes (fresh)
• 1 oz (30g) diced onion
• 1 oz (30g) diced zucchini
• 1 oz (30g) diced mushrooms
• 1 clove garlic, minced
• 1 tsp dried oregano
• 1 tsp dried basil
• 1/2 tsp paprika
• 1/2 tsp salt
• 1/4 tsp black pepper
• 2 oz (60g) mozzarella cheese (optional)
• Cooking spray

Instructions:

1. Preheat your air fryer to 375°F (190°C).

2. Cut the tops off the bell peppers and remove the seeds and membranes from the inside, creating a hollow space for the stuffing.

3. In a large skillet over medium heat, cook the ground turkey until it's browned and fully cooked. Drain any excess fat if necessary.

4. Add the diced onions, zucchini, mushrooms, and minced garlic to the skillet with the cooked turkey. Sauté the mixture for 3-4 minutes until the vegetables soften.

5. Stir in the cooked rice, diced tomatoes, dried oregano, dried basil, paprika, salt, and black pepper. Mix everything together until well combined.

6. Stuff each bell pepper with the ground turkey and rice mixture. Press the filling down gently to ensure they are tightly packed.

7. If desired, sprinkle shredded mozzarella cheese on top of each stuffed pepper.

8. Lightly coat the air fryer basket with cooking spray to prevent sticking.

9. Place the stuffed peppers in the air fryer basket, making sure they are stable and not tipping over.

10. Air fry the stuffed peppers at 375°F (190°C) for 15-20 minutes or until the peppers are tender and the filling is heated through. Cooking times may vary depending on the size and thickness of the peppers.

11. Once the stuffed peppers are done, carefully remove them from the air fryer using tongs or a spatula.

12. Let the stuffed peppers cool slightly before serving.

13. Serve the Air Fryer Stuffed Peppers with Ground Turkey as a wholesome and satisfying meal.

Nutritional values:
Calories: 270 kcal | Fat: 8g | Saturated Fat: 2g | Trans Fat: 0g | Cholesterol: 46mg | Sodium: 400mg | Carbohydrates: 30g | Fiber: 5g | Sugars: 6g | Protein: 21g

Air Fryer Mediterranean Stuffed Mushrooms

Serving: 4 | Preparation time: 10 minutes | Cooking time: 10-12 minutes

Ingredients:
- 8 oz (240g) mushrooms, cleaned and stems removed
- 2 oz (60g) hummus
- 0.8 oz (20g) crumbled feta cheese
- 4 oz (40g) sun-dried tomatoes, chopped
- 0.8 oz (20g) chopped Kalamata olives
- 1 oz (30g) chopped fresh parsley
- 1/4 tsp garlic powder
- Salt and pepper to taste
- Cooking spray

Instructions:

1. Preheat the air fryer to 360°F (182°C).

2. In a mixing bowl, combine the hummus, crumbled feta cheese, chopped sun-dried tomatoes, chopped Kalamata olives, chopped fresh parsley, garlic powder, and salt and pepper to taste.

3. Mix well until everything is evenly combined.

4. Stuff each mushroom cap with the mixture and place them in the air fryer basket.

5. Lightly spray the stuffed mushrooms with cooking spray.

6. Cook for 10-12 minutes or until the mushrooms are tender and the filling is golden brown.

7. Remove the mushrooms from the air fryer and serve hot.

Nutritional values:
Calories: 74 kcal | Fat: 4g | Protein: 3g | Carbs: 7g | Net carbs: 5g | Fiber: 2g | Cholesterol: 7mg | Sodium: 232mg | Potassium: 296mg

Air Fryer Lentil Meatballs with Marinara Sauce

Serving: 4 | Preparation Time: 30 minutes

Ingredients:
- 7 oz (200g) cooked lentils
- 2 oz (60g) low-carb breadcrumbs
- 2 oz (60g) grated vegan Parmesan cheese
- 2 tbsp tomato paste
- 2 cloves garlic, minced
- 1 tsp dried oregano
- 1 tsp dried basil
- Cooking spray
- 1/2 tsp onion powder
- 1/2 tsp salt
- 1/4 tsp black pepper
- 8 oz (240g) marinara sauce

Instructions:

1. In a food processor, combine the cooked lentils, breadcrumbs, vegan Parmesan cheese, tomato paste, minced garlic, dried oregano, dried basil, onion powder, salt, and black pepper. Pulse until well combined and the mixture holds together.

2. Shape the lentil mixture into meatball-sized balls, using about 1-2 tablespoons of the mixture for each meatball. Place them on a plate or tray.

3. Preheat the air fryer to 375°F (190°C).

4. Lightly grease the air fryer basket with cooking spray or olive oil to prevent sticking.

5. Place the lentil meatballs in a single layer in the air fryer basket, making sure they don't touch each other.

6. Air fry the meatballs for 15-18 minutes, shaking the basket or flipping the meatballs halfway through the cooking time, until they are crispy and golden brown on the outside.

7. While the meatballs are cooking, heat the marinara sauce in a small saucepan over low heat until warmed through.

8. Once the lentil meatballs are cooked, remove them from the air fryer and serve them with the warm marinara sauce.

Note: These lentil meatballs are a delicious and nutritious alternative to traditional meat-based meatballs. They are packed with protein from lentils and are full of flavor from the herbs and spices. Serve them as an appetizer, over pasta, or in a sandwich for a satisfying meal.

Nutritional values:
Calories: 150kcal | Fat: 2g | Protein: 8g | Carbs: 26g | Fiber: 6g | Sugar: 2g | Sodium: 340mg

Air Fryer Sausage Stuffed Mushrooms

Serving: 4 | Preparation Time: 25 minutes

Ingredients:

• 10 oz (300g) cremini or button mushrooms
• 4 oz (115g) Italian sausage, casings removed
• 0.8 oz (25g) grated Parmesan cheese
• 2 cloves garlic, minced
• 1 tbsp olive oil

• 1/2 tsp dried oregano
• 1/4 tsp salt
• 1/4 tsp black pepper
• Fresh parsley, chopped (for garnish)

Instructions:

1. Preheat the air fryer to 375°F (190°C).

2. Remove the stems from the mushrooms and set aside. Place the mushroom caps on a plate.

3. In a skillet over medium heat, cook the Italian sausage, breaking it into crumbles, until browned and cooked through. Remove from heat and let it cool slightly.

4. In a bowl, combine the cooked sausage, grated Parmesan cheese, minced garlic, olive oil, dried oregano, salt, and black pepper. Mix well.

5. Spoon the sausage mixture into each mushroom cap, filling them generously.

6. Place the stuffed mushrooms in the air fryer basket in a single layer, making sure they are not overcrowded.

7. Cook for 10-12 minutes until the mushrooms are tender and the sausage is nicely browned.

8. Remove the stuffed mushrooms from the air fryer and garnish with freshly chopped parsley.

9. Allow them to cool slightly before serving.

Note: These air fryer sausage-stuffed mushrooms make a delicious appetizer or side dish. The combination of Italian sausage and Parmesan cheese creates a flavorful filling. You can adjust the seasoning and add your favorite herbs or spices to customize the taste.

Nutritional values:
Calories: 140kcal | Fat: 10g | Protein: 8g | Carbs: 3g | Fiber: 1g | Sugar: 1g | Sodium: 280mg | Potassium: 270mg

Air Fryer Crab Cakes with Remoulade Sauce

Serving: 4 | Preparation Time: 20 minutes

Ingredients:

• 7.5 oz (225g) lump crab meat
• 1 oz (30g) low-carb breadcrumbs
• 2 oz (60g) low fat Greek yougurt
• 1 tbsp Dijon mustard

- 1 tbsp Worcestershire sauce (make sure it's sugar free)
- 1 oz (30g) green onion, finely chopped
- 1/2 tsp Old Bay seasoning
- 1/4 tsp salt

Remoulade Sauce Ingredients:
- 2 oz (60g) low fat Greek yougurt
- 1 tbsp Dijon mustard
- 1 tbsp lemon juice
- 1 tbsp capers, chopped
- 1 tbsp fresh parsley, chopped
- 1/2 tsp paprika
- 1/4 tsp cayenne pepper (optional)

Instructions:
1. Preheat the air fryer to 375°F (190°C).
2. In a medium bowl, gently combine the lump crab meat, breadcrumbs, low fat Greek yougurt, Dijon mustard, Worcestershire sauce, green onion, Old Bay seasoning, and salt. Be careful not to break up the crab meat too much.
3. Form the mixture into 4 equal-sized crab cakes and place them in the air fryer basket.
4. Cook the crab cakes in the air fryer for 10-12 minutes, or until golden brown and crispy.
5. While the crab cakes are cooking, prepare the remoulade sauce. In a small bowl, whisk together the low fat Greek yougurt, Dijon mustard, lemon juice, capers, fresh parsley, paprika, and cayenne pepper (if desired).
6. Serve the air fryer crab cakes hot with a dollop of remoulade sauce on top.

Note: The remoulade sauce adds a tangy and creamy element to complement the crab cakes. Enjoy them as a tasty addition to your meal.

Nutritional values:
Calories: 250kcal | Fat: 20g | Protein: 12g | Carbs: 6g | Fiber: 1g | Sugar: 1g | Sodium: 740mg | Potassium: 240mg

Air Fryer Bacon Wrapped Jalapeno Poppers

Serving: 4 | Preparation Time: 25 minutes

Ingredients:
- 3 oz (90g) jalapeno peppers
- 4 oz (115g) cream cheese
- 1 oz (30g) shredded cheddar cheese
- 4 oz (115g) bacon

Instructions:
1. Preheat the air fryer to 400°F (200°C).
2. Cut the jalapeno peppers in half lengthwise and remove the seeds and membranes using a spoon.
3. In a bowl, combine the cream cheese and shredded cheddar cheese.
4. Fill each jalapeno half with the cheese mixture.
5. Wrap each stuffed jalapeno half with a slice of bacon, securing it with toothpicks if necessary.
6. Place the bacon-wrapped jalapeno poppers in the air fryer basket in a single layer, making sure they are not touching each other.
7. Cook for 12-15 minutes, or until the bacon is crispy and the peppers are tender.
8. Carefully remove the jalapeno poppers from the air fryer and let them cool for a few minutes before serving.

Note: These air fryer bacon-wrapped jalapeno poppers are a popular appetizer that combines spicy jalapeno peppers, creamy cheese filling, and crispy bacon. They are perfect for parties or game nights. Adjust the spice level by removing or keeping the jalapeno seeds and membranes. Be cautious while handling jalapenos and avoid touching your face or eyes.

Nutritional values:
Calories: 120kcal | Fat: 10g | Protein: 4g | Carbs: 2g | Fiber: 0g | Sugar: 1g | Sodium: 220mg | Potassium: 100mg

Air Fryer Buffalo Chicken Meatballs with Blue Cheese Dressing

Serving: 4 | Preparation Time: 25 minutes

Ingredients:

For the Buffalo Chicken Meatballs:
- 15 oz (450g) ground chicken

- 1 oz (30g) low-carb breadcrumbs
- 2 oz (60ml) melted butter
- 1 egg, beaten
- 1 tsp garlic powder
- 1/2 tsp onion powder
- 1/2 tsp salt
- 1/4 tsp black pepper

For the Blue Cheese Dressing:
- 4 oz (120g) low fat Greek yougurt
- 2 oz (60g) sour cream
- 1 oz (30ml) milk
- 2 oz (55g) crumbled blue cheese
- 1 tbsp lemon juice
- 1/2 tsp garlic powder
- Salt and pepper to taste

Instructions:

1. Preheat the air fryer to 375°F (190°C).

2. In a large bowl, combine the ground chicken, breadcrumbs, melted butter, beaten egg, garlic powder, onion powder, salt, and black pepper. Mix well until all the ingredients are evenly incorporated.

3. Shape the mixture into bite-sized meatballs and place them in the air fryer basket.

4. Cook the meatballs in the air fryer for 15-18 minutes, or until they are cooked through and browned.

5. While the meatballs are cooking, prepare the blue cheese dressing. In a bowl, whisk together the sour cream, Greak yougurt milk, crumbled blue cheese, lemon juice, garlic powder, salt, and pepper until well combined.

6. Once the meatballs are done, remove them from the air fryer and let them cool for a few minutes.

7. Serve the Buffalo chicken meatballs with the blue cheese dressing on the side for dipping.

Note: These air fryer Buffalo chicken meatballs are a spicy and flavorful appetizer or party snack. The combination of ground chicken, hot sauce, and melted butter creates a classic Buffalo flavor. The blue cheese dressing adds a creamy and tangy element to complement the heat.

Nutritional values:
Calories: 180kcal | Fat: 11g | Protein: 15g | Carbs: 4g | Fiber: 0g | Sugar: 1g | Sodium: 490mg | Potassium: 270mg

Air Fryer Mushroom and Swiss Cheese Sliders

Serving: 8 | Preparation Time: 20 minutes

Ingredients:
- 8 oz (240g) slider whole-wheat buns
- 7.5 oz (225g) mushrooms, sliced
- 1 oz (30g) onion, thinly sliced
- 2 tbsp olive oil
- 1 garlic clove, minced
- Salt and pepper to taste
- 4 oz (120g) Swiss cheese slices
- Mustard, for serving (optional)

Instructions:

1. Preheat the air fryer to 375°F (190°C).

2. In a skillet, heat the olive oil over medium heat. Add the sliced mushrooms, onion, minced garlic, salt, and pepper. Cook until the mushrooms and onions are softened and golden brown, about 5-7 minutes.

3. Slice the slider buns in half horizontally. Place the bottom halves of the buns in the air fryer basket.

4. Spoon the cooked mushroom and onion mixture onto the bottom halves of the buns, spreading it evenly.

5. Top each slider with a small Swiss cheese slice.

6. Place the top halves of the buns on top of the cheese slices.

7. Transfer the air fryer basket to the air fryer and cook for 5-7 minutes, or until the cheese is melted and the sliders are warmed through.

8. Remove the sliders from the air fryer and let them cool slightly.

9. Serve the mushroom and Swiss cheese sliders with mustard on the side, if desired.

Note: These air fryer mushroom and Swiss cheese sliders are a delicious and easy-to-make appetizer or light meal. The sautéed mushrooms and onions provide a savory and earthy flavor, while the melted Swiss cheese adds a creamy and melty goodness. Customize the sliders with your favorite condiments and enjoy!

Nutritional values:
Calories: 240kcal | Fat: 12g | Protein: 8g | Carbs: 25g | Fiber: 2g | Sugar: 4g | Sodium: 300mg | Potassium: 200mg

Air Fryer Sweet and Spicy Chicken Drumsticks

Serving: 4 | Preparation Time: 35 minutes (including marinating time)

Ingredients:
- 30 oz (900g) chicken drumsticks
- 2 oz (60ml) less sodium soy sauce
- 2 tsp honey
- 1 tsp minced garlic
- Salt and pepper to taste
- Sesame seeds and chopped green onions for garnish

Instructions:
1. Preheat the air fryer to 400°F (200°C).
2. In a bowl, whisk together the soy sauce, honey, minced garlic, salt, and pepper to make the marinade.
3. Place the chicken drumsticks in a large ziplock bag or a bowl. Pour the marinade over the drumsticks, ensuring each piece is coated. Marinate in the refrigerator for at least 30 minutes, or overnight for more flavor.
4. Remove the drumsticks from the marinade and shake off any excess.
5. Place the drumsticks in a single layer in the air fryer basket. You may need to cook them in batches depending on the size of your air fryer.
6. Cook the drumsticks in the air fryer for 25-30 minutes, flipping halfway through, until they are golden brown and cooked through. The internal temperature should reach 165°F (74°C).
7. Once the drumsticks are done, remove them from the air fryer and let them cool for a few minutes.
8. Garnish the drumsticks with sesame seeds and chopped green onions before serving.

Note: The use of too much sugar or honey might affect your sugar level, be careful of excess sugar or honey

Nutritional values:
Calories: 280kcal | Fat: 14g | Protein: 24g | Carbs: 14g | Fiber: 0g | Sugar: 12g | Sodium: 1200mg | Potassium: 300mg

Air Fryer Italian Sausage and Peppers

Serving: 4 | Preparation Time: 20 minutes

Ingredients:
- 3 oz (90g) Italian sausages
- 4 oz (120g) bell peppers, sliced
- 2 oz (60g) onion, sliced
- 2 cloves garlic, minced
- 2 tbsp olive oil
- 1 tsp Italian seasoning
- 1/2 tsp paprika
- 1/4 tsp red pepper flakes (adjust to taste)
- Salt and pepper to taste
- Cooking spray

Instructions:
1. Preheat the air fryer to 400°F (200°C).
2. In a large bowl, combine the sliced bell peppers, onion, minced garlic, olive oil, Italian seasoning, paprika, red pepper flakes, salt, and pepper. Toss well to coat the vegetables with the seasonings.
3. Spray the air fryer basket with cooking spray.
4. Place the Italian sausages and seasoned vegetables in the air fryer basket, arranging them in a single layer.
5. Cook for 15-20 minutes, shaking the basket or flipping the sausages halfway through, until the sausages are cooked through and the vegetables are tender and slightly charred.
6. Once cooked, remove the Italian sausages and peppers from the air fryer.
7. Serve hot with your choice of side dishes or as a filling for sandwiches or wraps.

Nutritional values:
Calories: 320kcal | Fat: 26g | Protein: 12g | Carbohydrates: 10g | Fiber: 3g | Cholesterol: 25mg | Sodium: 500mg | Potassium: 450mg

Air Fryer Prosciutto-Wrapped Melon

Serving: 4 | Preparation Time: 10 minutes | Cooking Time: 8 minutes

Ingredients:

- 3 oz (90g) of prosciutto
- 10 oz (300g) cubes of ripe cantaloupe or honeydew melon
- Fresh mint leaves, for garnish
- Cooking spray

Instructions:

1. Preheat the air fryer to 400°F (200°C).
2. Take a slice of prosciutto and place a cube of melon at one end.
3. Roll the prosciutto tightly around the melon cube and secure with a toothpick.
4. Repeat the process with the remaining prosciutto slices and melon cubes.
5. Lightly spray the air fryer basket with cooking spray to prevent sticking.
6. Place the prosciutto-wrapped melon in a single layer in the air fryer basket.
7. Cook in the air fryer at 400°F (200°C) for 6-8 minutes, or until the prosciutto is crispy.
8. Remove the prosciutto-wrapped melon from the air fryer and let cool slightly.
9. Garnish with fresh mint leaves, if desired.
10. Serve as an appetizer or snack.

Nutritional values:

Calories: 100kcal | Fat: 5g | Protein: 8g | Carbohydrates: 7g | Fiber: 1g | Cholesterol: 20mg | Sodium: 700mg | Potassium: 250mg

Air Fryer Bacon-Wrapped Pineapple Bites

Serving: 4 | Preparation Time: 15 minutes | Cooking Time: 10 minutes

Ingredients:

- 3 oz (90 g) slices of bacon
- 6 oz (180g) 16 pineapple chunks (fresh or canned)
- Wooden toothpicks
- Cooking spray

Instructions:

1. Preheat the air fryer to 400°F (200°C).
2. Cut each bacon slice in half lengthwise to create thinner strips.
3. Take a bacon strip and wrap it around a pineapple chunk. Secure the bacon with a toothpick.
4. Repeat the process with the remaining bacon and pineapple chunks.
5. Lightly spray the air fryer basket with cooking spray to prevent sticking.
6. Place the bacon-wrapped pineapple bites in a single layer in the air fryer basket.
7. Cook in the air fryer at 400°F (200°C) for 8-10 minutes, or until the bacon is crispy.
8. Remove the bacon-wrapped pineapple bites from the air fryer and let cool slightly.
9. Serve as an appetizer or party snack.

Nutritional values:

Calories: 120kcal | Fat: 8g | Protein: 4g | Carbohydrates: 9g | Fiber: 1g | Cholesterol: 15mg | Sodium: 280mg | Potassium: 110mg

Air Fryer Korean BBQ Beef Skewers

Serving: 4 | Preparation Time: 20 minutes | Cooking Time: 10 minutes

Ingredients:

- 15 oz (450g) beef sirloin, thinly sliced
- 2 oz (60g) less sodium soy sauce
- 2 tsp honey
- 2 tbsp sesame oil
- 2 cloves garlic, minced
- 1 tbsp grated fresh ginger
- 1 tbsp rice vinegar
- 1 tbsp gochujang (Korean red pepper paste)
- 1 tbsp sesame seeds
- 4 oz (120 g) green onions, sliced
- Wooden skewers, soaked in water for 30 minutes
- Cooking spray

Instructions:

1. In a bowl, combine soy sauce, honey, sesame oil, minced garlic, grated ginger, rice vinegar, gochujang, sesame seeds, and sliced green onions. Mix well to make the marinade.

2. Add the thinly sliced beef to the marinade and toss to coat. Let it marinate for at least 10 minutes, or refrigerate for up to 4 hours for better flavor.

3. Preheat the air fryer to 400°F (200°C).

4. Thread the marinated beef slices onto the soaked wooden skewers, folding them back and forth in a zigzag pattern.

5. Lightly spray the air fryer basket with cooking spray to prevent sticking.

6. Place the beef skewers in a single layer in the air fryer basket.

7. Cook in the air fryer at 400°F (200°C) for 8-10 minutes, flipping halfway through, until the beef is cooked to your desired doneness and nicely charred.

8. Remove the skewers from the air fryer and let them rest for a few minutes.

9. Serve the Air Fryer Korean BBQ Beef Skewers hot as an appetizer or main dish. They can be enjoyed on their own or with steamed rice and a side of kimchi.

Note: The use of too much sugar or honey might affect your sugar level, be careful of excess sugar or honey

Nutritional values:
Calories: 280kcal | Fat: 16g | Protein: 26g | Carbohydrates: 9g | Fiber: 1g | Cholesterol: 70mg | Sodium: 1100mg | Potassium: 470mg

Air Fryer Mini Quiches

Serving: 4 | Preparation Time: 15 minutes | Cooking Time: 15 minutes

Ingredients:
- 4 large eggs
- 2 oz (60ml) milk
- 2 oz (60g) shredded cheddar cheese
- 1 oz (30g) diced ham or cooked bacon
- 1 oz (30g) diced bell peppers
- 1 oz (30g) diced onions
- Salt and pepper to taste
- Cooking spray

Instructions:

1. Preheat the air fryer to 375°F (190°C).

2. In a bowl, whisk the eggs and milk together until well combined.

3. Add the shredded cheddar cheese, diced ham or bacon, diced bell peppers, and diced onions to the egg mixture. Season with salt and pepper to taste. Stir to combine.

4. Lightly spray the air fryer basket or individual silicone muffin cups with cooking spray to prevent sticking.

5. Pour the egg mixture evenly into the muffin cups, filling each cup about two-thirds full.

6. Place the filled muffin cups in the air fryer basket, leaving some space between them.

7. Cook in the air fryer at 375°F (190°C) for 12-15 minutes or until the quiches are set and golden brown on top.

8. Remove the mini quiches from the air fryer and let them cool slightly before serving.

9. Serve the Air Fryer Mini Quiches as a delightful snack, or brunch option.

Nutritional values:
Calories: 130kcal | Fat: 9g | Protein: 8g | Carbohydrates: 3g | Fiber: 0g | Cholesterol: 185mg | Sodium: 220mg | Potassium: 105mg

Chapter 10.
Sauces and dressings

Garlic Aioli

Serving: 4 | Prep time: 5 minutes | Cook time: 5 minutes

Ingredients:

· 4 oz (113 g) plain Greek yogurt
· 2 cloves garlic, minced
· 1 tbsp lemon juice
· 1/4 tsp Dijon mustard
· 1/4 tsp salt
· 1/4 tsp black pepper
· 1 tbsp olive oil
· 1 tbsp water

Directions:

1. In a small bowl, combine Greek yogurt, minced garlic, lemon juice, Dijon mustard, salt, and black pepper.
2. Slowly drizzle in olive oil while stirring continuously to emulsify the mixture.
3. If the aioli is too thick, add water gradually until desired consistency is reached.
4. Refrigerate for at least 30 minutes before serving to allow flavors to meld.

Useful Tip: To control sugar intake, always opt for plain Greek yogurt without added sugars. Check labels for hidden sugars in condiments like mustard.

Nutritional values: Calories: 40 kcal | Fat: 3 g | Protein: 2 g | Carbs: 2 g | Net carbs: 1 g | Fiber: 1 g | Cholesterol: 0 mg | Sodium: 150 mg | Potassium: 30 mg

Cilantro Lime Dressing

Serving: 4 | Prep time: 5 minutes | Cook time: 5 minutes

Ingredients:

· 2 oz (57 g) fresh cilantro leaves
· 2 cloves garlic
· 1/4 cup olive oil
· 2 tbsp lime juice
· 1/4 tsp salt
· 1/4 tsp black pepper
· 2 tbsp water
· 1 tsp honey (optional, for sweetness)

Directions:

1. In a food processor, combine cilantro leaves, garlic, olive oil, lime juice, salt, and black pepper.
2. Pulse until the mixture is well blended and smooth.
3. Add water gradually until desired consistency is achieved.
4. Taste and adjust seasoning if necessary. If you prefer a sweeter taste, you can add honey at this stage.

Useful Tip: Always check the labels for added sugars, especially in ingredients like honey, to ensure it aligns with your dietary needs.

Nutritional values: Calories: 110 kcal | Fat: 12 g | Protein: 0 g | Carbs: 1 g | Net carbs: 1 g | Fiber: 0 g | Cholesterol: 0 mg | Sodium: 150 mg | Potassium: 20 mg

BBQ Sauce

Serving: 4 | Prep time: 5 minutes | Cook time: 5 minutes

Ingredients:

· 4 oz (113 g) tomato paste
· 2 tbsp apple cider vinegar
· 1 tbsp Worcestershire sauce (choose a low-sugar variety)
· 1 tbsp low-sodium soy sauce
· 1 tbsp Dijon mustard
· 1/2 tsp smoked paprika
· 1/4 tsp garlic powder
· 1/4 tsp black pepper

Directions:

1. In a bowl, whisk together tomato paste, apple cider vinegar, Worcestershire sauce, soy sauce, Dijon mustard, smoked paprika, garlic powder, and black pepper until well combined.
2. Taste and adjust seasoning if needed, adding more vinegar for acidity or more paprika for smokiness.
3. If the sauce is too thick, thin it out with a bit of water, one tablespoon at a time, until desired consistency is reached.

Useful Tip: When selecting Worcestershire sauce and soy sauce, look for varieties labeled "low-sodium" or "reduced-sodium" to minimize sodium intake.

Nutritional values: Calories: 25 kcal | Fat: 0 g | Protein: 1 g | Carbs: 5 g | Net carbs: 4 g | Fiber: 1 g | Cholesterol: 0 mg | Sodium: 150 mg | Potassium: 200 mg

Lemon Herb Butter Sauce

Serving: 4 | Prep time: 5 minutes | Cook time: 5 minutes

Ingredients:

· 4 tbsp unsalted butter
· 2 cloves garlic, minced
· Zest of 1 lemon
· 2 tbsp lemon juice
· 1 tbsp fresh parsley, finely chopped
· 1 tbsp fresh chives, finely chopped
· 1/4 tsp salt
· 1/4 tsp black pepper

Directions:

1. In a small saucepan over low heat, melt the unsalted butter.
2. Add minced garlic and cook for 1-2 minutes until fragrant.
3. Stir in lemon zest, lemon juice, fresh parsley, fresh chives, salt, and black pepper.
4. Cook for another 1-2 minutes, stirring constantly, until the herbs are wilted and flavors are combined.

Useful Tip: Opt for unsalted butter to control sodium intake, and always check the label for added sugars in lemon juice.

Nutritional values: Calories: 100 kcal | Fat: 11 g | Protein: 0 g | Carbs: 1 g | Net carbs: 1 g | Fiber: 0 g | Cholesterol: 30 mg | Sodium: 75 mg | Potassium: 20 mg

Creamy Avocado Dressing

Serving: 4 | Prep time: 5 minutes | Cook time: 5 minutes

Ingredients:

· 1 ripe avocado, peeled and pitted
· 2 oz (60 ml) plain Greek yogurt
· 2 tbsp lemon juice
· 1 clove garlic, minced
· 2 tbsp water
· 1/4 tsp salt
· 1/4 tsp black pepper
· 1 tbsp fresh cilantro, chopped

Directions:

1. In a blender or food processor, combine the ripe avocado, plain Greek yogurt, lemon juice, minced garlic, water, salt, and black pepper.
2. Blend until smooth and creamy, scraping down the sides as needed to ensure all ingredients are well combined.
3. Add fresh cilantro to the mixture and pulse briefly until incorporated.
4. If the dressing is too thick, add additional water, one tablespoon at a time, until desired consistency is reached.

Useful Tip: To prevent oxidation, store any leftover dressing in an airtight container with plastic wrap pressed directly onto the surface of the dressing.

Nutritional values: Calories: 70 kcal | Fat: 5 g | Protein: 3 g | Carbs: 5 g | Net carbs: 2 g | Fiber: 3 g | Cholesterol: 0 mg | Sodium: 150 mg | Potassium: 260 mg

Tahini Sauce

Serving: 4 | Prep time: 5 minutes | Cook time: 5 minutes

Ingredients:

· 4 tbsp tahini
· 2 tbsp lemon juice
· 2 cloves garlic, minced

- 2 tbsp water
- 1/4 tsp salt
- 1/4 tsp black pepper
- 1 tbsp extra virgin olive oil
- 1 tbsp fresh parsley, chopped

Directions:

1. In a small bowl, combine tahini, lemon juice, minced garlic, water, salt, and black pepper.
2. Whisk the ingredients together until smooth and well incorporated.
3. Drizzle in the extra virgin olive oil while whisking continuously to emulsify the sauce.
4. Add fresh parsley to the mixture and stir until evenly distributed.

Useful Tip: If the tahini sauce is too thick, gradually add more water until you reach your desired consistency.

Nutritional values: Calories: 100 kcal | Fat: 9 g | Protein: 2 g | Carbs: 4 g | Net carbs: 3 g | Fiber: 1 g | Cholesterol: 0 mg | Sodium: 150 mg | Potassium: 80 mg

Teriyaki Sauce

Serving: 4 | Prep time: 5 minutes | Cook time: 10 minutes

Ingredients:

- 3 tbsp low-sodium soy sauce
- 2 tbsp water
- 2 tbsp rice vinegar
- 2 cloves garlic, minced
- 1 tbsp fresh ginger, grated
- 1 tbsp sesame oil
- 1 tbsp erythritol (or preferred sugar substitute)
- 1/4 tsp black pepper

Directions:

1. In a small bowl, combine low-sodium soy sauce, water, rice vinegar, minced garlic, grated ginger, sesame oil, erythritol, and black pepper.
2. Whisk the ingredients together until well combined.
3. Transfer the mixture to a saucepan and cook over medium heat for 5-7 minutes, stirring occasionally, until slightly thickened.
4. Remove from heat and let cool before serving.

Useful Tip: Taste the sauce before serving and adjust sweetness or saltiness according to your preference, keeping in mind to use sugar substitutes for a diabetic-friendly option.

Nutritional values: Calories: 35 kcal | Fat: 3 g | Protein: 1 g | Carbs: 2 g | Net carbs: 1 g | Fiber: 1 g | Cholesterol: 0 mg | Sodium: 250 mg | Potassium: 50 mg

Dijon Mustard Dressing

Serving: 4 | Prep time: 5 minutes | Cook time: 5 minutes

Ingredients:

- 3 tbsp olive oil
- 2 tbsp Dijon mustard
- 1 tbsp lemon juice
- 1 clove garlic, minced
- 1/4 tsp dried thyme
- 1/4 tsp dried parsley
- Salt and pepper, to taste

Directions:

1. In a small bowl, whisk together olive oil, Dijon mustard, lemon juice, minced garlic, dried thyme, and dried parsley until well combined.
2. Season with salt and pepper according to taste preferences.
3. Adjust the consistency by adding more olive oil if desired.

Useful Tip: Store any leftover dressing in an airtight container in the refrigerator for up to one week. Before using, let it come to room temperature and shake well to re-emulsify.

Nutritional values: Calories: 120 kcal | Fat: 14 g | Protein: 0 g | Carbs: 1 g | Net carbs: 1 g | Fiber: 0 g | Cholesterol: 0 mg | Sodium: 80 mg | Potassium: 20 mg

Balsamic Glaze

Serving: 4 | Prep time: 2 minutes | Cook time: 20 minutes

Ingredients:

- 8 oz (240 ml) balsamic vinegar
- 1 tbsp olive oil
- 1 clove garlic, minced

- 1/2 tsp dried thyme
- 1/2 tsp dried rosemary
- Salt and pepper, to taste

Directions:

1. In a small saucepan, combine balsamic vinegar, olive oil, minced garlic, dried thyme, and dried rosemary.
2. Bring the mixture to a boil over medium-high heat, then reduce the heat to low and let it simmer for about 20 minutes or until it thickens and reduces by half, stirring occasionally.
3. Once the glaze reaches a syrupy consistency, remove it from the heat and season with salt and pepper according to taste.
4. Let the glaze cool slightly before serving.

Useful Tip: Be cautious when reducing the balsamic vinegar as it can easily burn due to its high sugar content. Keep an eye on it and adjust the heat as needed.

Nutritional values: Calories: 40 kcal | Fat: 2 g | Protein: 0 g | Carbs: 5 g | Net carbs: 5 g | Fiber: 0 g | Cholesterol: 0 mg | Sodium: 10 mg | Potassium: 20 mg

Honey Mustard Sauce

Serving: 4 | Prep time: 2 minutes | Cook time: 5 minutes

Ingredients:

- 3 tbsp Dijon mustard
- 2 tsp honey
- 1 tbsp apple cider vinegar
- 1/2 tbsp olive oil
- 1/4 tsp garlic powder
- Salt and pepper, to taste

Directions:

1. In a small bowl, whisk together Dijon mustard, honey, apple cider vinegar, olive oil, and garlic powder until well combined.
2. Season with salt and pepper according to taste preference.
3. Adjust the consistency by adding more olive oil for a thinner sauce or more mustard for a thicker consistency, if desired.

Useful Tip: Ensure to use sugar-free honey to keep the sauce low in carbohydrates. Always check the labels for hidden sugars in condiments like mustard and honey.

Nutritional values: Calories: 40 kcal | Fat: 2 g | Protein: 0 g | Carbs: 6 g | Net carbs: 6 g | Fiber: 0 g | Cholesterol: 0 mg | Sodium: 170 mg | Potassium: 5 mg

Mayonnaise

Serving: 4 | Prep time: 5 minutes | Cook time: 5 minutes

Ingredients:

- 2 large egg yolks
- 1 tsp Dijon mustard
- 1/2 tsp apple cider vinegar
- 4 oz (120 ml) olive oil
- 1/2 tsp lemon juice
- Salt and pepper, to taste

Directions:

1. In a mixing bowl, whisk together the egg yolks, Dijon mustard, and apple cider vinegar until well combined.
2. Gradually drizzle in the olive oil while continuing to whisk vigorously until the mixture starts to thicken.
3. Once thickened, add lemon juice, salt, and pepper, and continue whisking until the mayonnaise reaches your desired consistency.

Useful Tip: Ensure all ingredients are at room temperature for optimal emulsification, and adjust the seasoning according to your taste preferences. Always check the labels for hidden sugars in condiments like mustard.

Nutritional values: Calories: 216 kcal | Fat: 24 g | Protein: 1 g | Carbs: 0 g | Net carbs: 0 g | Fiber: 0 g | Cholesterol: 92 mg | Sodium: 11 mg | Potassium: 8 mg

Ketchup

Serving: 4 | Prep time: 5 minutes | Cook time: 20 minutes

Ingredients:

- 10 oz (280 g) tomatoes, chopped
- 2 oz (60 ml) tomato paste
- 2 cloves garlic, minced

- 1 tbsp apple cider vinegar
- 1/2 tsp onion powder
- 1/4 tsp smoked paprika
- 1/4 tsp salt
- 1/4 tsp black pepper

Directions:

1. In a saucepan, combine the chopped tomatoes, tomato paste, minced garlic, apple cider vinegar, onion powder, smoked paprika, salt, and black pepper.
2. Bring the mixture to a gentle simmer over medium heat.
3. Reduce the heat to low and let it simmer uncovered for about 15-20 minutes, stirring occasionally, until the tomatoes break down and the mixture thickens.
4. Remove the saucepan from the heat and let the ketchup cool slightly.
5. Transfer the mixture to a blender or food processor and blend until smooth.

Useful Tip: Store the ketchup in an airtight container in the refrigerator for up to one week. Adjust the seasoning according to your taste preferences.

Nutritional values: Calories: 31 kcal | Fat: 0.5 g | Protein: 1 g | Carbs: 6 g | Net carbs: 4 g | Fiber: 2 g | Cholesterol: 0 mg | Sodium: 166 mg | Potassium: 271 mg

Chapter 11. Desserts

Air Fryer Cinnamon Apples

Serving: 4 | Preparation time: 10 minutes | Cooking time: 8-10 minutes

Ingredients:

- 15 oz (450g) apples, peeled and sliced
- 2 tsp cinnamon
- 1 tsp stevia or any non-sugar sweetener to your test
- 1 tbsp lemon juice
- 1 tbsp melted butter or coconut oil (for vegan option)

Instructions:

1. In a large bowl, toss together the sliced apples, cinnamon, stevia or any non-sugar sweetener, lemon juice, and melted butter or coconut oil.
2. Transfer the apple mixture to an air fryer-safe container.
3. Preheat the air fryer to 375°F (190°C).
4. Place the container in the air fryer basket and cook for 8-10 minutes, shaking the container every 3 minutes, or until the apples are tender and lightly browned.
5. Remove the container from the air fryer and let the apples cool for a few minutes before serving.

Note: The use of too much sugar or honey might affect your sugar level, be careful of excess sugar or honey

Nutritional values:

Calories: 120 kcal | Fat: 3g | Protein: 1g | Carbs: 25g | Net carbs: 19g | Fiber: 6g | Cholesterol: 8mg | Sodium: 29mg | Potassium: 239mg

Air Fryer Chocolate Chip Cookies

Serving: 4 | Preparation time: 20 minutes | Cooking time: 6-8 minutes

Ingredients:

- 3.5 oz (100g) unsalted butter, at room temperature
- 2 oz (60g) stevia or any non-sugar sweetener to your test
- 1 large egg
- 1 tsp vanilla extract
- 4 oz (120g) almond flour
- 1/2 tsp baking soda
- 1/4 tsp salt
- 1 oz (30g) semisweet chocolate chips

Instructions:

1. In a large mixing bowl, cream together the butter, stevia or any non-sugar sweetener until light and fluffy.
2. Add the egg and vanilla extract and beat until well combined.
3. In a separate mixing bowl, whisk together the flour, baking soda, and salt.
4. Gradually add the dry ingredients to the wet ingredients, mixing until just combined.
5. Fold in the chocolate chips.
6. Preheat the air fryer to 350°F (180°C).
7. Drop spoonful's of cookie dough onto an air fryer-safe tray or basket, leaving about 2 inches between each cookie.
8. Cook the cookies for 6-8 minutes, or until lightly golden brown.
9. Remove the cookies from the air fryer and let them cool on a wire rack.

Note: The use of too much sugar or honey might affect your sugar level, be careful of excess sugar or honey

Nutritional values:

Calories: 139 kcal | Fat: 6g | Protein: 2g | Carbs: 20g | Net carbs: 18g | Fiber: 2g | Cholesterol: 20mg | Sodium: 57mg | Potassium: 96mg

Air Fryer Chocolate Cake

Serving: 4 | Preparation time: 10 minutes | Cooking time: 12-15 minutes

Ingredients:

- 1 oz (30g) almond flour
- 2 tbsp unsweetened cocoa powder
- 1/4 tsp baking powder
- Pinch of salt
- 2 oz (60ml) unsweetened almond milk
- 1 tsp maple syrup
- 1 tbsp melted coconut oil
- 1/2 tsp vanilla extract

Instructions:

1. In a medium bowl, whisk together the flour, cocoa powder, baking powder, and salt.
2. In another bowl, whisk together the almond milk, maple syrup, melted coconut oil, and vanilla extract.
3. Pour the wet ingredients into the dry ingredients and stir until well combined.
4. Pour the batter into an 4-inch cake pan that fits in your air fryer.
5. Preheat the air fryer to 350°F (175°C).
6. Place the cake pan in the air fryer basket and cook for 12-15 minutes or until a toothpick inserted into the center comes out clean.
7. Remove the cake pan from the air fryer and let the cake cool in the pan for 5 minutes before removing it from the pan.

Nutritional values:

Calories: 228 kcal | Fat: 11g | Protein: 4g | Carbs: 30g | Net carbs: 23g | Fiber: 7g | Cholesterol: 0mg | Sodium: 56mg | Potassium: 314mg

Air Fryer Blueberry Muffins

Serving: 4 | Preparation time: 10 minutes | Cooking time: 12-15 minutes

Ingredients:

- 4 oz (120g) almond flour
- 3.5 oz (100g) stevia or any non-sugar sweetener to your test
- 1 tsp baking powder
- 1/4 tsp salt
- 2 oz (60ml) vegetable oil
- 1 large egg
- 1/2 tsp vanilla extracts
- 2.5 oz (75g) fresh blueberries
- 2 oz (60ml) milk
- Cooking spray

Instructions:

1. In a medium mixing bowl, whisk together the flour, stevia or any non-sugar sweetener to your test, baking powder, and salt.
2. In a separate small mixing bowl, whisk together the vegeta ble oil, milk, egg, and vanilla extract.
3. Add the wet ingredients to the dry ingredients and stir until just combined.
4. Gently fold in the blueberries.
5. Preheat the air fryer to 325°F (160°C).
6. Grease 4 muffin cups with cooking spray and divide the batter evenly among them.
7. Place the muffin cups in the air fryer basket and cook for 12-15 minutes or until a toothpick inserted into the center of a muffin comes out clean.
8. Once done, remove the muffin cups from the air fryer and let cool for a few minutes.
9. Gently remove the muffins from the cups and serve warm or at room temperature.

Note: The use of too much sugar or honey might affect your sugar level, be careful of excess sugar or honey

Nutritional values:

Calories: 275 kcal | Fat: 11g | Protein: 4g | Carbs: 41g | Net carbs: 38g | Fiber: 3g | Cholesterol: 47mg | Sodium: 167mg | Potassium: 95mg

Air Fryer Banana Bread

Serving: 4 | Preparation time: 10 minutes | Cooking time: 25-30 minutes

Ingredients:

- 4 oz (120g) 2 ripe bananas, mashed
- 2 oz (60ml) vegetable oil
- 1.8 oz (50g) stevia or any non-sugar sweetener to your test
- 1 tsp vanilla extracts
- 4 oz (125g) almond flour
- 1/2 tsp baking soda

- 1/4 tsp salt
- 1/2 tsp ground cinnamon
- 0.88 oz (25g) chopped walnuts (optional)
- Cooking spray

Instructions:

1. Preheat the air fryer to 300°F (150°C).
2. In a large mixing bowl, combine the mashed bananas, vegetable oil, stevia or any non-sugar sweetener to your test, and vanilla extract.
3. In a separate mixing bowl, whisk together the flour, baking soda, salt, and ground cinnamon.
4. Gradually add the dry ingredients to the wet ingredients and mix until just combined.
5. Fold in the chopped walnuts (if using).
6. Grease a small loaf pan with cooking spray and pour the batter into the pan.
7. Place the loaf pan in the air fryer basket and cook for 25-30 minutes or until a toothpick inserted in the center comes out clean.
8. Once done, remove the banana bread from the air fryer and let it cool for a few minutes before slicing and serving.
9. Enjoy!

Note: The use of too much sugar or honey might affect your sugar level, be careful of excess sugar or honey

Nutritional values:

Calories: 210 kcal | Fat: 10g | Protein: 2g | Carbs: 29g | Net carbs: 26g | Fiber: 3g | Cholesterol: 0mg | Sodium: 130mg | Potassium: 164mg

Air Fryer Carrot Cake Cupcakes

Serving: 4 | Preparation time: 10 minutes | Cooking time: 15-20 minutes

Ingredients:

- 4 oz (120g) almond flour
- 1 oz (30g) coconut flour
- 1 tsp baking powder
- 1/2 tsp baking soda
- 1 tsp ground cinnamon
- 1/4 tsp ground nutmeg
- 1/4 tsp salt
- 1 oz (30g) Carrots grated

- Cooking spray

Instructions:

1. Preheat the air fryer to 350°F (175°C).
2. In a mixing bowl, combine the almond flour, coconut flour, baking powder, baking soda, ground cinnamon, ground nutmeg, and salt. Mix well.
3. Add the grated carrots to the dry mixture and stir until evenly distributed.
4. Line the cupcake molds or silicone liners with cupcake liners or lightly grease them with cooking spray.
5. Spoon the carrot cake batter into the prepared cupcake molds, filling each about 2/3 full.
6. Place the filled cupcake molds into the preheated air fryer basket, making sure they are spaced apart for even cooking.
7. Cook the carrot cake cupcakes in the air fryer at 350°F (175°C) for 15-20 minutes or until a toothpick inserted into the center comes out clean.
8. Once cooked, carefully remove the cupcakes from the air fryer and let them cool completely before serving.
9. Optionally, you can frost the cooled cupcakes with cream cheese frosting or dust them with powdered sugar.

Nutritional values:

Calories: 314 kcal | Fat: 24g | Protein: 7g | Carbs: 18g | Net carbs: 8g | Fiber: 10g | Cholesterol: 93mg | Sodium: 366mg | Potassium: 322mg

Air Fryer Lemon Bars

Serving: 4 | Preparation time: 10 minutes | Cooking time: 15-20 minutes

Ingredients:

- 4 oz (120g) almond flour
- 3 tbsp melted butter
- 1 tsp maple syrup
- 2 eggs
- 4 oz (120ml) freshly squeezed lemon juice
- Zest of 1 lemon
- 1 oz (30g) coconut flour
- 1/4 tsp baking powder
- Pinch of salt

Instructions:

1. Preheat the air fryer to 325°F (165°C).
2. In a mixing bowl, combine almond flour, melted butter, and maple syrup. Mix until crumbly.
3. Press the mixture into the bottom of a greased 8x8 inch baking dish.
4. In another mixing bowl, beat the eggs and add lemon juice and lemon zest. Mix well.
5. In a separate bowl, whisk together coconut flour, baking powder, and salt.
6. Add the dry ingredients to the wet ingredients and mix well.
7. Pour the lemon filling over the crust.
8. Place the baking dish in the air fryer basket and cook for 15-20 minutes, or until the edges start to turn golden brown and the filling is set.
9. Let the lemon bars cool completely before slicing and serving.

Note: The use of too much sugar or honey might affect your sugar level, be careful of excess sugar or honey

Nutritional values:

Calories: 186 kcal | Fat: 14g | Protein: 5g | Carbs: 10g | Net carbs: 6g | Fiber: 4g | Cholesterol: 71mg | Sodium: 46mg | Potassium: 112mg

Air Fryer Peanut Butter Cookies

Serving: 4 | Preparation time: 10 minutes | Cooking time: 8-10 minutes

Ingredients:

- 4.2 oz (128g) creamy peanut butter
- 1 oz (30ml) maple syrup
- 1 egg
- 1/2 tsp vanilla extract
- 1/2 tsp baking powder
- 1/4 tsp salt
- 1 oz (32g) coconut flour

Instructions:

1. Preheat the air fryer to 325°F (165°C).
2. In a mixing bowl, combine peanut butter, maple syrup, egg, and vanilla extract. Mix well.
3. Add baking powder, salt, and coconut flour to the mixture and mix until dough forms.

4. Roll the dough into 12 balls and place them on a parchment-lined air fryer basket.
5. Flatten each ball with a fork to create a criss-cross pattern.
6. Place the basket in the air fryer and cook for 8-10 minutes, or until the cookies are golden brown and crispy.
7. Remove the cookies from the air fryer and let them cool completely before serving.

Nutritional values:

Calories: 95 kcal | Fat: 7g | Protein: 3g | Carbs: 6g | Net carbs: 3g | Fiber: 3g | Cholesterol: 20mg | Sodium: 101mg | Potassium: 104mg

Air Fryer Pumpkin Spice Donuts

Serving: 4 | Preparation time: 15 minutes | Cooking time: 10-12 minutes

Ingredients:

- 4 oz (120g) almond flour
- 4 oz (120g) pumpkin puree
- 2 Eggs
- Sweetener of choice
- 2 oz (60ml) melted coconut oil
- 1 tsp baking powder
- 1 tsp ground cinnamon
- 1/4 tsp ground nutmeg
- 2 oz (60ml) Almond milk

Instructions:

1. Preheat the air fryer to 350°F (175°C).
2. In a mixing bowl, whisk together almond flour, sweetener, baking powder, and spices.
3. In another bowl, whisk together almond milk, pumpkin puree, eggs, and melted coconut oil.
4. Add the wet ingredients to the dry ingredients and mix until smooth.
5. Transfer the batter to a piping bag or a ziplock bag with a corner snipped off.
6. Pipe the batter into a greased donut mold, filling each mold about 2/3 full.
7. Place the mold in the air fryer and cook for 10-12 minutes, or until the donuts are lightly golden and cooked through.

8. Remove the mold from the air fryer and let the donuts cool for a few minutes before removing them from the mold.

9. Repeat with the remaining batter, if needed.

Nutritional values:

Calories: 149 kcal | Fat: 12g | Protein: 4g | Carbs: 7g | Net carbs: 4g | Fiber: 3g | Cholesterol: 16mg | Sodium: 52mg | Potassium: 118mg

Air Fryer Chocolate Covered Strawberries

Serving | Preparation time: 10 minutes | Cooking time: 4-6 minutes

Ingredients:

• 5 oz (150g) dark chocolate chips
• 15 oz (450g) fresh strawberries, washed and dried

Instructions:

1. Preheat the air fryer to 320°F (160°C).

2. Place the dark chocolate chips in a microwave-safe bowl and melt them in the microwave in 30-second intervals, stirring in between, until fully melted and smooth.

3. Hold a strawberry by the stem and dip it into the melted chocolate, coating it about three-quarters of the way up.

4. Gently shake off any excess chocolate and place the chocolate-covered strawberry on a parchment-lined air fryer basket.

5. Repeat the process with the remaining strawberries.

6. Place the basket in the air fryer and cook for 4-6 minutes, or until the chocolate is set.

7. Remove the basket from the air fryer and let the strawberries cool completely before serving.

Nutritional values:

Calories: 79 kcal | Fat: 5g | Protein: 1g | Carbs: 8g | Net carbs: 6g | Fiber: 2g | Cholesterol: 0mg | Sodium: 1mg | Potassium: 97mg

Air Fryer Almond Butter Cookies

Serving: 4 | Preparation time: 15 minutes | Cooking time: 8-10 minutes

Ingredients:

• 4 oz (120g) almond flour

• 4 oz (120g) almond butter
•1 oz (30ml) maple syrup
• 1 egg
• 1 tsp vanilla extract
• 1/2 tsp baking powder
• 1/4 tsp salt

Instructions:

1. Preheat the air fryer to 350°F (175°C).

2. In a mixing bowl, combine the almond flour, baking powder, and salt.

3. Add the almond butter, maple syrup, egg, and vanilla extract. Mix until well combined.

4. Form the dough into small balls and flatten slightly onto a piece of parchment paper.

5. Place the parchment paper with the cookie dough onto the air fryer basket.

6. Air fryer the cookies at 350°F (175°C) for 8-10 minutes, or until golden brown.

7. Remove the basket from the air fryer and let the cookies cool on the parchment paper for a few minutes before serving.

Nutritional values:

Calories: 152 kcal | Fat: 11g | Protein: 5g | Carbs: 11g | Net carbs: 9g | Fiber: 2g | Cholesterol: 21mg | Sodium: 72mg | Potassium: 130mg

Air Fryer Peach Cobbler

Serving: 4 | Preparation time: 10 minutes | Cooking time: 12-15 minutes

Ingredients:

• 15 oz (450g) peaches, peeled and sliced
• 2 oz (60g) almond flour
• 1 oz (30g) coconut flour
• 2 oz (60ml) melted coconut oil
• 1 tsp maple syrup
• 1 tsp baking powder
• 1/2 tsp cinnamon
• Pinch of salt

Instructions:

1. Preheat the air fryer to 350°F (175°C).

2. In a mixing bowl, combine the almond flour, coconut flour, baking powder, cinnamon, and salt.

3. Add the melted coconut oil and maple syrup to the bowl and mix well to form a crumbly dough.

4. Arrange the peach slices in a single layer in a baking dish that fits in the air fryer basket.

5. Sprinkle the dough over the peaches in an even layer.

6. Place the baking dish in the air fryer basket and air fry at 350°F (175°C) for 12-15 minutes, or until the topping is golden brown and the peaches are tender.

7. Remove the baking dish from the air fryer and let the cobbler cool for a few minutes before serving.

Nutritional values:

Calories: 243 kcal | Fat: 20g | Protein: 3g | Carbs: 14g | Net carbs: 9g | Fiber: 5g | Cholesterol: 0mg | Sodium: 63mg | Potassium: 213mg

Air Fryer Chocolate Brownies

Serving: 4 | Preparation time: 10 minutes | Cooking time: 12-15 minutes

Ingredients:

• 2 oz (60g) almond flour
• 0.70 oz (20g) cocoa powder
• 2 oz (60ml) melted coconut oil
• 1 tsp maple syrup
• 1 tsp baking powder
• Pinch of salt
• 2 large eggs
• 1 tsp Coconut oil

Instructions:

1. Preheat the air fryer to 325°F (160°C).

2. In a mixing bowl, combine the almond flour, cocoa powder, baking powder, and salt.

3. Add the melted coconut oil, maple syrup, and eggs to the bowl and mix well to form a smooth batter.

4. Grease a small baking dish that fits in the air fryer basket with some coconut oil.

5. Pour the batter into the baking dish and smooth out the surface.

6. Place the baking dish in the air fryer basket and air fry at 325°F (160°C) for 12-15 minutes, or until a toothpick inserted in the center comes out clean.

7. Remove the baking dish from the air fryer and let the brownies cool for a few minutes before slicing and serving.

Nutritional values:

Calories: 316 kcal | Fat: 28g | Protein: 7g | Carbs: 13g | Net carbs: 9g | Fiber: 4g | Cholesterol: 93mg | Sodium: 84mg | Potassium: 215mg

Air Fryer Raspberry Cheesecake

Serving: 4 | Preparation time: 15 minutes | Cooking time: 20-25 minutes

Ingredients:

• 2 oz (60g) almond flour
• 0.8 oz (25g) coconut flour
• 2 oz (60ml) melted coconut oil
• 1 tsp maple syrup
• 1 tsp vanilla extract
• Pinch of salt
• 8 oz (225g) cream cheese, softened
• 1.4 oz (40g) raspberries

Instructions:

1. Preheat the air fryer to 325°F (160°C).

2. In a mixing bowl, combine the almond flour, coconut flour, melted coconut oil, maple syrup, vanilla extract, and salt.

3. Press the mixture into the bottom of a small cheesecake pan that fits in the air fryer basket.

4. In a separate mixing bowl, beat the cream cheese until smooth.

5. Add the raspberries to the bowl and beat until well combined.

6. Pour the cream cheese mixture over the crust in the cheesecake pan and smooth out the surface.

7. Place the cheesecake pan in the air fryer basket and air fry at 325°F (160°C) for 20-25 minutes, or until the cheesecake is set.

8. Remove the cheesecake pan from the air fryer and let it cool for a few minutes before removing it from the pan.

9. Chill the cheesecake in the fridge for at least an hour before serving.

Nutritional values:

Calories: 329 kcal | Fat: 32g | Protein: 6g | Carbs: 8g | Net carbs: 4g | Fiber: 4g | Cholesterol: 69mg | Sodium: 170mg | Potassium: 104mg

Air Fryer Mini Cherry Pies

Serving: 4 | Preparation time: 15 minutes | Cooking time: 10-12 minutes

Ingredients:

- 4 oz (125g) almond flour
- 2 oz (60ml) melted coconut oil
- 1 tsp maple syrup
- 1/4 tsp almond extract
- 1/4 tsp salt
- 1.8 oz (75g) pitted cherries, halved
- 1 tbsp stevia or any non-sugar sweetener to your test
- 1/4 tsp ground cinnamon

Instructions:

1. Preheat the air fryer to 350°F (180°C).
2. In a mixing bowl, combine the almond flour, melted coconut oil, maple syrup, almond extract, and salt.
3. Divide the dough into 4 equal parts and shape them into mini pie crusts that fit into a muffin tin.
4. In another mixing bowl, combine the cherries, stevia or any non-sugar sweetener to your test, and ground cinnamon.
5. Fill the mini pie crusts with the cherry mixture.
6. Place the mini cherry pies in the air fryer basket and air fry at 350°F (180°C) for 10-12 minutes, or until the crust is golden brown.
7. Remove the mini cherry pies from the air fryer and let them cool for a few minutes before removing them from the muffin tin.
8. Serve warm or chilled.

Nutritional values:

Calories: 288 kcal | Fat: 25g | Protein: 5g | Carbs: 13g | Net carbs: 7g | Fiber: 6g | Cholesterol: 0mg | Sodium: 151mg | Potassium: 134mg

Air Fryer Chocolate Covered Pretzels

Serving: 4 | Preparation time: 10 minutes | Cooking time: 2-3 minutes

Ingredients:

- 3.5 oz (100g) pretzel sticks
- 3 oz (90g) sugar-free chocolate chips
- 1 tsp coconut oil

Instructions:

1. Preheat the air fryer to 320°F (160°C).
2. Line a baking sheet with parchment paper.
3. In a microwave-safe bowl, melt the sugar-free chocolate chips and coconut oil in 30-second intervals until smooth and creamy.
4. Dip each pretzel stick into the melted chocolate and coat it evenly.
5. Place the chocolate-covered pretzels on the prepared baking sheet.
6. Place the baking sheet with the chocolate-covered pretzels in the air fryer basket and air fry at 320°F (160°C) for 2-3 minutes or until the chocolate has hardened.
7. Remove the chocolate-covered pretzels from the air fryer and let them cool for a few minutes before serving.

Nutritional values:

Calories: 120 kcal | Fat: 5g | Protein: 2g | Carbs: 19g | Net carbs: 14g | Fiber: 5g | Cholesterol: 0mg | Sodium: 190mg | Potassium: 50mg

Air Fryer Peanut Butter Cupcakes

Serving: 4 | Preparation time: 15 minutes | Cooking time: 10-12 minutes

Ingredients:

- 2 oz (60g) almond flour
- 1.2 oz (32g) coconut flour
- 2 oz (64g) natural peanut butter
- 2 oz (60ml) unsweetened almond milk
- 1 oz (30ml) keto-friendly maple syrup
- 2 large eggs
- 1 tsp vanilla extract

Instructions:

1. Preheat the air fryer to 320°F (160°C).
2. In a mixing bowl, combine almond flour, coconut flour, natural peanut butter, unsweetened almond milk, keto-friendly maple syrup, eggs, and vanilla extract. Mix well until a smooth batter forms.
3. Line a muffin tin with liners and pour the batter into each muffin liner, filling them 2/3 full.

4. Place the muffin tin in the air fryer basket and air fry at 320°F (160°C) for 10-12 minutes or until a toothpick inserted in the center comes out clean.

5. Remove the muffin tin from the air fryer and let the cupcakes cool in the tin for 5 minutes before transferring them to a wire rack to cool completely.

6. Serve and enjoy.

Nutritional values:

Calories: 160 kcal | Fat: 11g | Protein: 6g | Carbs: 10g | Net carbs: 4g | Fiber: 6g | Cholesterol: 55mg | Sodium: 80mg | Potassium: 110mg

Air Fryer Lemon Pound Cake

Serving: 4 | Preparation time: 15 minutes | Cooking time: 30-35 minutes

Ingredients:

- 6 oz (180g) almond flour
- 1 oz (28g) coconut flour
- 3 large eggs
- 2 oz (60ml) fresh lemon juice
- 1 tbsp lemon zest
- 1/4 tsp salt
- 1 tsp vanilla extract
- 1 tsp baking powder
- 4 oz (120g) unsalted butter, softened
- 1 oz (30ml) keto-friendly maple syrup

Instructions:

1. Preheat the air fryer to 320°F (160°C).

2. In a mixing bowl, cream together the softened unsalted butter and keto-friendly maple syrup until light and fluffy.

3. Add in the eggs one at a time, mixing well after each addition.

4. Stir in the fresh lemon juice, lemon zest, and vanilla extract.

5. In a separate bowl, mix together the almond flour, coconut flour, baking powder, and salt.

6. Gradually add the dry mixture to the wet mixture, mixing well until a smooth batter forms.

7. Pour the batter into a greased 6-inch (15cm) cake pan.

8. Place the cake pan in the air fryer basket and air fry at 320°F (160°C) for 30-35 minutes or until a toothpick inserted in the center comes out clean.

9. Remove the cake pan from the air fryer and let the cake cool in the pan for 5-10 minutes before transferring it to a wire rack to cool completely.

Nutritional values:

Calories: 260 kcal | Fat: 23g | Protein: 6g | Carbs: 11g | Net carbs: 5g | Fiber: 6g | Cholesterol: 100mg | Sodium: 140mg | Potassium: 100mg

Air Fryer Apple Turnovers

Serving: 4 | Preparation time: 15 minutes | Cooking time: 10-12 minutes

Ingredients:

- 7 oz (200g) apple, peeled, cored, and chopped
- 1 tbsp lemon juice
- 1 tbsp stevia or any non-sugar sweetener to your test
- 1/2 tsp ground cinnamon
- 1/8 tsp ground nutmeg
- 1 sheet filo pastry, thawed
- 1 egg, beaten
- 1 tbsp stevia or any non-sugar sweetener

Instructions:

1. In a bowl, mix together the chopped apple, lemon juice, 1 tablespoon of stevia or any non-sugar sweetener, cinnamon, and nutmeg.

2. Cut the filo pastry sheet into 4 squares.

3. Place a heaping tablespoon of the apple mixture in the center of each filo pastry square.

4. Brush the edges of each square with beaten egg and fold in half to create a triangle.

5. Use a fork to press down the edges and seal the turnover.

6. Brush the tops of the turnovers with beaten egg and sprinkle with stevia or any non-sugar sweetener.

7. Preheat the air fryer to 375°F (190°C).

8. Place the turnovers in the air fryer basket and air fry at 375°F (190°C) for 10-12 minutes or until golden brown.

9. Remove the turnovers from the air fryer and let them cool for a few minutes before serving.

Note: The use of too much sugar or honey might affect your sugar level, be careful of excess sugar or honey

Nutritional values:

Calories: 255 kcal | Fat: 14g | Protein: 4g | Carbs: 29g | Net carbs: 24g | Fiber: 5g | Cholesterol: 31mg | Sodium: 157mg | Potassium: 141mg

Air Fryer Caramelized Bananas

Serving: 4 | Preparation time: 10 minutes | Cooking time: 5-6 minutes

Ingredients:

• 8 oz (240g) bananas
• 2 tbsp unsalted butter or coconut oil
• 2 tsp sugar-free maple syrup
• 1/4 tsp ground cinnamon
• Pinch of salt

Instructions:

1. Preheat the air fryer to 375°F (190°C).
2. Peel the bananas and cut them into 1/2 inch (1.25cm) slices.
3. Melt the unsalted butter or coconut oil in a microwave-safe bowl or on the stovetop.
4. Add the sugar-free maple syrup, ground cinnamon, and a pinch of salt to the melted butter or coconut oil, and mix until combined.
5. Add the sliced bananas to the mixture and toss to coat evenly.
6. Place the coated banana slices in the air fryer basket in a single layer.
7. Air fry the banana slices at 375°F (190°C) for 5-6 minutes, flipping halfway through.
8. Once done, remove the air fryer basket and let the caramelized bananas cool for a few minutes before serving.

Nutritional values:

Calories: 156 kcal | Fat: 10g | Protein: 1g | Carbs: 18g | Net carbs: 13g | Fiber: 5g | Cholesterol: 23mg | Sodium: 40mg | Potassium: 222mg

Air Fryer Mixed Berry Crisp

Serving: 4 | Preparation time: 10 minutes | Cooking time: 12-15 minutes

Ingredients:

• 9 oz (280g) mixed frozen berries
• 1 oz (30g) almond flour
• 1 tsp sugar-free maple syrup
• 1/4 tsp ground cinnamon
• Pinch of salt
• 1 oz (30g) chopped pecans
• 2 tbsp unsalted butter or coconut oil, melted

Instructions:

1. Preheat the air fryer to 375°F (190°C).
2. In a mixing bowl, combine the mixed frozen berries, almond flour, melted unsalted butter or coconut oil, sugar-free maple syrup, ground cinnamon, and a pinch of salt. Toss to combine.
3. Transfer the berry mixture into a small baking dish that fits inside the air fryer basket. If desired, sprinkle chopped pecans over the top of the mixture.
4. Place the baking dish in the air fryer basket and air fry at 375°F (190°C) for 12-15 minutes or until the top is golden brown and the berries are bubbling.
5. Once done, remove the baking dish from the air fryer and let cool for a few minutes before serving.

Note: To make this recipe vegan, substitute the unsalted butter with coconut oil. The use of too much sugar or honey might affect your sugar level, be careful of excess sugar or honey

Nutritional values:

Calories: 203 kcal | Fat: 18g | Protein: 3g | Carbs: 11g | Net carbs: 7g | Fiber: 4g | Cholesterol: 23mg | Sodium: 29mg | Potassium: 150mg

Air Fryer Vanilla Cupcakes

Serving: 4 | Preparation time: 10 minutes | Cooking time: 12-15 minutes

Ingredients:

• 2 oz (60g) almond flour
• 1 oz (28g) coconut flour
• 2 tbsp flaxseed meal
• 2 oz (60ml) unsweetened almond milk
• 2 tbsp unsalted butter or coconut oil, melted
• 2 large eggs

- 2 tsp vanilla extract
- 1.5 oz (48g) erythritol or sweetener of choice
- 1 tsp baking powder

Instructions:

1. Preheat the air fryer to 320°F (160°C).
2. In a mixing bowl, whisk together the almond flour, coconut flour, flaxseed meal, and baking powder.
3. In a separate bowl, beat together the melted unsalted butter or coconut oil, eggs, unsweetened almond milk, vanilla extract, and erythritol until well combined.
4. Add the dry ingredients to the wet ingredients and whisk until smooth.
5. Line a muffin tin with four paper liners and divide the batter evenly between them.
6. Place the muffin tin in the air fryer basket and air fry at 320°F (160°C) for 12-15 minutes or until a toothpick inserted into the center of a cupcake comes out clean.
7. Once done, remove the muffin tin from the air fryer and let cool for a few minutes before serving.

Nutritional values:

Calories: 200 kcal | Fat: 16g | Protein: 6g | Carbs: 8g | Net carbs: 3g | Fiber: 5g | Cholesterol: 118mg | Sodium: 180mg | Potassium: 90mg

Air Fryer Strawberry Shortcake

Serving: 4 | Preparation time: 10 minutes | Cooking time: 10-12 minutes

Ingredients:

- 4 oz (120g) almond flour
- 2 tbsp coconut flour
- 2 tbsp sugar-free maple syrup
- 1/4 tsp baking powder
- 1/4 tsp salt
- 1 large egg
- 1 tsp vanilla extracts
- 1/2 sliced strawberries
- Whipped cream, for serving
- 2 tbsp unsalted butter or coconut oil, melted

Instructions:

1. Preheat the air fryer to 320°F (160°C).

2. In a mixing bowl, combine the almond flour, coconut flour, baking powder, and salt.
3. Add the melted unsalted butter or coconut oil, sugar-free maple syrup, egg, and vanilla extract to the dry mixture, and mix until well combined.
4. Fold in the sliced strawberries.
5. Scoop the batter into silicone cupcake liners or a greased ramekin, filling them about 3/4 full.
6. Place the cupcake liners or ramekin in the air fryer basket and air fry at 320°F (160°C) for 10-12 minutes, or until the shortcakes are lightly golden on top and cooked through.
7. Once done, remove the air fryer basket and let the shortcakes cool for a few minutes before serving.
8. Cut the shortcakes in half, and top each half with whipped cream and additional sliced strawberries, if desired.

Nutritional values:

Calories: 268 kcal | Fat: 23g | Protein: 7g | Carbs: 11g | Net carbs: 6g | Fiber: 5g | Cholesterol: 62mg | Sodium: 162mg | Potassium: 130mg

Air Fryer Coconut Macaroons

Serving: 4 | Preparation time: 10 minutes | Cooking time: 10-12 minutes

Ingredients:

- 5 oz (160g) unsweetened shredded coconut
- 1/2 tsp vanilla extract
- 4 oz (120ml) sweetened condensed milk
- 1/4 tsp almond extract
- 2 large egg whites
- Pinch of salt

Instructions:

1. Preheat the air fryer to 325°F (165°C).
2. In a mixing bowl, combine the shredded coconut, sweetened condensed milk, vanilla extract, and almond extract. Mix until well combined.
3. In a separate bowl, beat the egg whites and salt until stiff peaks form.
4. Gently fold the beaten egg whites into the coconut mixture until evenly incorporated.
5. Using a small cookie scoop or tablespoon, scoop the mixture and drop onto a parchment-lined air fryer basket.

6. Place the basket in the air fryer and cook for 10-12 minutes, or until the macaroons turn golden brown.

7. Remove the macaroons from the air fryer and let them cool completely.

8. Serve the air fryer coconut macaroons chilled.

Nutritional values:

Calories: 92 kcal | Fat: 6g | Protein: 1g | Carbs: 8g | Net carbs: 7g | Fiber: 1g | Sugar: 7g | Sodium: 43mg | Potassium: 66mg

Air Fryer Pear Crisp

Serving: 4 | Preparation time: 10 minutes | Cooking time: 10-12 minutes

Ingredients:

For the Filling:

• 4 oz (120g) ripe pears, peeled, cored, and slice

• 2 tbsp stevia or any non-sugar sweetener to your test

• 1 tbsp lemon juice

• 1 tsp ground cinnamon

For the Crisp Topping:

• 2 oz (60g) old-fashioned rolled oats

• 2 oz (60g) almond flour

• 2 tbsp stevia or any non-sugar sweetener to your test

• 1/4 tsp ground cinnamon

• 2 tbsp unsalted butter, cold and cut into small pieces

• Pinch of salt

• Optional Toppings:

• Vanilla ice cream or whipped cream

Instructions:

1. Preheat your air fryer to 350°F (175°C).

2. In a large mixing bowl, combine the sliced pears, stevia or any non-sugar sweetener, lemon juice, and ground cinnamon. Toss everything together until the pears are evenly coated. Set the bowl aside.

3. In a separate bowl, prepare the crisp topping. Mix together the rolled oats, almond flour, stevia or any non-sugar sweetener, cold butter pieces, ground cinnamon, and a pinch of salt. Using your fingers or a fork, work the butter into the dry ingredients until the mixture resembles coarse crumbs.

4. Take an oven-safe dish or a small baking pan that fits into your air fryer basket. Transfer the prepared pear filling into the dish, spreading it out evenly.

5. Sprinkle the crisp topping over the pear filling, covering it entirely with the mixture.

6. Place the dish with the pear crisp into the pre-heated air fryer basket.

7. Air fry the pear crisp at 350°F (175°C) for about 15-20 minutes, or until the pears are tender and the crisp topping turns golden brown and crunchy.

8. Once the pear crisp is done, remove it from the air fryer and let it cool slightly.

9. Serve the Air Fryer Pear Crisp warm. You can enjoy it as is or add a scoop of vanilla ice cream or a dollop of whipped cream on top for extra indulgence.

Nutritional values:

Calories: 190 kcal | Fat: 7g | Saturated Fat: 4g | Trans Fat: 0g | Cholesterol: 15mg | Sodium: 20mg | Carbohydrates: 34g | Fiber: 5g | Sugars: 18g | Protein: 2g

Chapter 12.
30 Days Meal Plan

MEAL PLAN WEEK 1

DAYS	BREAKFAST	LUNCH	SNACK	DINNER
Monday	Air Fryer Cinnamon Apple Oatmeal pg. 30	Air Fryer Grilled Chicken Salad pg. 32	Greek yogurt with berries	Air Fryer Beef Stir Fry pg. 76
Tuesday	Air Fryer Mushroom and Swiss Cheese Sliders pg. 113	Air Fryer Beef Meatballs pg. 75	Carrot sticks with hummus	Air Fryer Tofu pg. 98
Wednesday	Air Fryer Egg Muffins pg. 21	Air Fryer Broccoli Cheddar Soup pg. 45	String cheese and a small apple	Air Fryer Moroccan Spiced Lamb Chops pg. 81
Thursday	Air Fryer Turkey Sausage and Egg Breakfast Pockets pg. 28	Air Fryer Butternut Squash Soup pg. 41	Handful of mixed nuts	Air Fryer Stuffed Squash pg. 103
Friday	Air Fryer Cinnamon Sweet Potato Fries pg. 104	Air Fryer Turkey Legs with Rosemary and Thyme pg. 55	Apple slices with almond butter	Air Fryer Crab Cakes with Remoulade Sauce pg. 111
Saturday	Air Fryer Ham and Cheese Breakfast Pockets pg. 29	Air Fryer Chicken Drumsticks with Ranch Seasoning pg. 63	Cottage cheese with cucumber slices	Air Fryer Apple Cider Glazed Pork Tenderloin pg. 72
Sunday	Air Fryer Breakfast Stuffed Peppers pg. 26	Air Fryer Rosemary and Lemon Pork Chops pg. 69	Raw almonds and a piece of fruit	Air Fryer Veggie Burger pg. 99

MEAL PLAN WEEK 2

DAYS	BREAKFAST	LUNCH	SNACK	DINNER
Monday	Air Fryer Cinnamon Apple Oatmeal pg. 30	Air Fryer Chicken Noodle Soup pg. 39	Mixed nuts	Air Fryer Lamb and Chickpea Stew pg. 80
Tuesday	Air Fryer Sausage and Egg Breakfast Sandwich pg. 27	Air Fryer Beef Meatballs pg. 75	Almonds	Air Fryer Beef and Vegetable Kabobs pg. 74
Wednesday	Air Fryer Spinach and Feta Breakfast Pockets pg. 24	Air Fryer Chicken Lettuce Wraps pg. 66	Apple slices with peanut butter	Air Fryer Coconut Shrimp pg. 92
Thursday	Air Fryer Baked Brie with Honey and Almonds pg. 51	Air Fryer Turkey Burgers pg. 54	Celery sticks with cream cheese	Air Fryer Garlic Butter Scallops pg. 92
Friday	Air Fryer Breakfast Casserole pg. 20	Air Fryer Chicken Shawarma pg. 64	String cheese	Air Fryer Moroccan Spiced Lamb Chops pg. 81
Saturday	Air Fryer Cinnamon French Toast Sticks pg. 23	Air Fryer Cajun Pork Chops pg. 72	Carrot sticks with hummus	Air Fryer Apple Cider Glazed Pork Tenderloin pg. 72
Sunday	Air Fryer Ham and Cheese Omelette pg. 22	Air Fryer Chicken Wings with Garlic Parmesan Sauce pg. 60	Baby carrots with ranch dressing	Air Fryer Stuffed Peppers with Ground Turkey pg. 109

MEAL PLAN WEEK 3

DAYS	BREAKFAST	LUNCH	SNACK	DINNER
Monday	Air Fryer Breakfast Stuffed Peppers pg. 26	Air Fryer Mediterranean Salad pg. 36	String cheese	Air Fryer Blackened Catfish pg. 85
Tuesday	Air Fryer Breakfast Bagel Sandwich pg. 31	Air Fryer Turkey Sausage Patties pg. 55	Celery with almond butter	Air Fryer Beef Stir Fry pg. 76
Wednesday	Air Fryer Turkey Sausage and Egg Breakfast Pockets pg. 28	Air Fryer Grilled Cheese Sandwich pg. 50	Baby carrots with ranch dressing	Air Fryer Lamb and Vegetable Skewers pg. 79
Thursday	Air Fryer Bacon and Egg Cups pg. 25	Air Fryer Greek Lamb Meatballs pg. 79	Handful of walnuts	Air Fryer Moroccan Spiced Lamb Chops pg. 81
Friday	Air Fryer Avocado Egg Boats pg. 22	Air Fryer Clam Chowder pg. 42	Cucumber slices with hummus	Air Fryer Mediterranean Fish pg. 88
Saturday	Air Fryer Sausage and Egg Breakfast Sandwich pg. 27	Air Fryer Sausage Stuffed Mushrooms pg. 111	Mixed nuts	Air Fryer Blackened Catfish pg. 85
Sunday	Air Fryer Egg Muffins pg. 21	Air Fryer Chicken Tortilla Soup pg. 43	Sugar-free jello	Air Fryer Stuffed Peppers with Ground Turkey pg. 109

MEAL PLAN WEEK 4

DAYS	BREAKFAST	LUNCH	SNACK	DINNER
Monday	Air Fryer Hash Brown Egg Nests pg. 27	Air Fryer Chicken Shawarma pg. 64	Greek yogurt with berries	Air Fryer Crab Rangoon pg. 96
Tuesday	Air Fryer Spinach and Feta Breakfast Pockets pg. 24	Air Fryer Beef Kofta Kebabs pg. 77	Carrot sticks with hummus	Air Fryer BBQ Beef Ribs pg. 76
Wednesday	Air Fryer Blueberry Muffins pg. 23	Air Fryer Turkey Fajitas pg. 57	Cottage cheese with cucumber slices	Air Fryer Blackened Catfish pg. 85
Thursday	Air Fryer Baked Eggs in Tomato Sauce pg. 25	Air Fryer Chicken Parmesan pg. 62	Raw almonds and a piece of fruit	Air Fryer Split Pea Soup pg. 40
Friday	Air Fryer Bacon and Egg Cups pg. 25	Air Fryer Honey Mustard Pork Tenderloin pg. 69	Apple slices with almond butter	Air Fryer Moroccan Spiced Lamb Chops pg. 81
Saturday	Air Fryer Breakfast Empanadas pg. 29	Air Fryer Cajun Shrimp and Sausage pg. 93	String cheese and a small apple	Air Fryer Broccoli Cheddar Soup pg. 45
Sunday	Air Fryer Smoked Salmon and Avocado Salad pg. 37	Air Fryer Turkey Slices with Balsamic Glaze pg. 59	Handful of mixed nuts	Air Fryer Beef and Vegetable Kabobs pg. 74

Chapter 13.
Cooking Temperatures of Vegetable

NO.	VEGETABLE	Cooking Temperature (°F)	Cooking Time (minutes)
1	Asparagus	360-380	6-10
2	Broccoli	350-375	8-12
3	Brussels Sprouts	375-400	12-15
4	Carrots	350-375	12-15
5	Cauliflower	360-380	10-15
6	Green Beans	360-380	8-12
7	Mushrooms	350-370	6-10
8	Bell Peppers	370-390	8-12
9	Zucchini	360-380	6-10
10	Sweet Potatoes	350-375	15-20
11	Spinach (Leaves)	325-350	3-5
12	Eggplant	360-380	10-15
13	Tomatoes (Cherry)	325-350	4-7

Remember to preheat your air fryer before cooking and monitor the vegetables closely, as cooking times may vary based on the size and thickness of the pieces. Adjust the temperatures and times accordingly to achieve your desired level of crispiness and doneness.

Conclusion

The Diabetic Air Fryer Cookbook for Beginners is more than just a collection of recipes. It is a comprehensive guide that empowers individuals with diabetes to take control of their health and enjoy delicious meals. Throughout this book, we have explored the challenges of managing diabetes while striving for a healthy and flavorful diet.

By following the recipes and tips provided, you have gained the tools and knowledge needed to make informed choices about your meals. From breakfast to dessert, this cookbook offers a wide range of options that cater to your dietary needs. Each recipe is carefully crafted to ensure it is both nutritious and delicious, while keeping your blood sugar levels in check. The expertise of a seasoned chef and nutritionist has been shared with you, providing valuable insights into the world of diabetic-friendly cooking. You have learned how to make the most of your air fryer, a versatile kitchen appliance that can transform your culinary creations.

With the Diabetic Air Fryer Cookbook for Beginners, you are not only managing your diabetes effectively but also embracing a healthier and more vibrant lifestyle. The journey doesn't end here, though. Armed with these newfound skills, you can continue to explore the limitless possibilities of diabetic-friendly cooking.

Remember, the key lies in balance, creativity, and making choices that support your well-being. By prioritizing your health and enjoying flavorful meals, you have discovered that managing diabetes does not mean compromising on taste or satisfaction.

Pause! Before You Proceed

Greetings, health enthusiasts,

As we come to the end of the *Diabetic Air Fryer Cookbook for Beginners*, I want to express my deepest gratitude to you, my fellow health enthusiasts. Thank you for embarking on this culinary journey with me. I truly hope that these pages have sparked inspiration and that each recipe has been a stepping stone on your path to healthier, more satisfying meals.

Every dish in this book is carefully crafted to support your dietary needs while delivering delicious flavors. Your health and enjoyment are at the heart of every recipe, making healthy eating a delightful experience.

Your feedback is invaluable. Every comment and suggestion helps shape future editions, ensuring they meet your needs and aspirations even better. This exchange between us goes beyond the pages — it's a collaboration that fosters continuous improvement and support.

As a token of my deep appreciation for choosing this guide, I am thrilled to offer you an exclusive bonus: ***Bonus Diabetic Cookbook with 100 Recipes***. This gift is reserved only for you, my dedicated readers. Click the link below to access this special bonus and continue your journey towards healthier living.

Access Your Special Bonus Here! https://diabeticairfryer.site/

If you have any questions, suggestions, or feedback,
please reach out via email at isabella.abrams@proton.me.
Your input is highly valued and will be deeply considered.

With heartfelt thanks and anticipation,

Isabella Abrams

Made in the USA
Middletown, DE
29 August 2024

60005656R00080